THE NEMECHEK PROTOCOL FOR AUTISM AND DEVELOPMENTAL DISORDERS

A HOW-TO GUIDE TO RESTORING NEUROLOGICAL FUNCTION

DR. PATRICK M. NEMECHEK, D.O.

JEAN R. NEMECHEK, J.D.

CONTENTS

MEDICAL DISCLAIMER

The information and the images contained within this publication are provided as an informational resource only, and are not to be used or relied on for any diagnostic or medical or treatment purposes.

This information is not intended to be patient education, and does not create any patient-physician relationship.

Please consult with a licensed healthcare practitioner to determine if any of these particular therapeutic approaches is appropriate for you or your child.

GLOSSARY

A SHORT GLOSSARY OF SCIENTIFIC TERMS

- **ALA, Alpha-Linolenic Acid** = An omega-3 fatty acid commonly supplemented in the form of nuts, flax, or chia.
- **Arachidonic Acid** = An omega-6 fatty acid that is part of the inflammation-producing process.
- **Autonomic Nervous System** = A large portion of the nervous system that regulates blood pressure, coordinates all organs (heart, intestines, bladder, etc.), controls inflammation, and regulates hormone production.
- **Bacterial Overgrowth** = Often used to refer to excessive bacterial growth within a segment of the intestinal tract. Less specific than the term SIBO which also implies a positive methane or hydrogen breath test or an abnormal quantification study from small intestinal aspirate.
- **CBI** = Cumulative Brain Injury. The cumulative damage that results from the residual defects remaining after improperly repaired physical, inflammatory, or metabolic damage.
- **Concussion** = A physical injury to the brain that results in persistent symptoms for several days. Also referred to as a minor traumatic brain injury or mTBI.

- **Cumulative Brain Injury** = The cumulative damage that results from the residual defects remaining after improperly repaired physical, inflammatory, or metabolic damage.
- **Cytokines, Anti-Inflammatory** = Chemicals released from white blood cells that decrease the inflammatory response.
- **Cytokines, Pro-Inflammatory** = Chemicals released from white blood cells that increase the inflammatory response.
- **Developmental Delay** = The slowing of the normal rate of neurological and emotional maturation of a child. Often the result of excessive inflammation, nutritional deficiencies, and improper neuron pruning.
- **Developmental Arrest** = The complete stoppage of neurological and emotional maturation of a child. Often the result of excessive inflammation, nutritional deficiencies, and improper neuron pruning.
- **DHA** = Docosahexaenoic acid (DHA) is an omega-3 fatty acid that is a primary structural component of the human brain, cerebral cortex, skin, and retina. Dietary sources include wild fish, fish oil, and meat from animals that feed on their natural food (e.g., grass fed beef).
- **Digestive Enzymes** = Supplements often provided to improve digestion and intestinal symptoms.
- **Dysbiosis** = Refers to a general disruption of normal microbial balance within the intestinal tract. Dysbiosis can refer to any segment of the intestinal tract (mouth, small intestine, or colon), and although usually implies bacteria, may also be used in regard to protozoan, fungi, or archaebacteria.
- **EPA** = Eicosapentaenoic acid (EPA) is an omega-3 fatty acid. Dietary sources include wild fish, fish oil, and meat from animals that feed on their natural food (e.g., grass fed beef).
- **EVOO** = Extra Virgin Olive Oil. EVOO is the highest

quality of olive oil and is considered to have favorable flavor characteristics. It contains oleic acid which is an omega-9 fatty acid.

- **Inflammation** = A normal response by the immune system to fight infection or repair damaged tissues. Excessive inflammation can lead to damaging effects in the body.
- **Intestinal Bacterial Overgrowth** = Often used when referring to the excessive presence of bacteria within the small intestine. These bacteria often originate in the colon (lower or large intestine) and abnormally migrate up to the small intestine.
- **Inulin** = A prebiotic fiber that is preferentially digested by the types of bacteria that normally inhabit the small intestine.
- **Linolenic Acid** = An omega-6 fatty acid that is part of the inflammation-producing process. Commonly found in plants and in high concentrations within a wide variety of cooking oils.
- **Microglia, M0** = These are a specialized form of white blood cells that live in the brain. They are often referred to as surveillance or pruning microglia.
- **Microglia, M1** - These are a specialized form of white blood cells that live in the brain. They promote inflammation and are part of the healthy repair process but can cause damage if they become primed.
- **Microglia, M2** - These are a specialized form of white blood cells that live in the brain. They shut off inflammation and are part of the healthy repair process.
- **Microglia, Primed** = These are microglia that permanently morph into M1-microglia and prevent the brain from fully repairing brain trauma. They also are a major source of inflammatory cytokines within the brain.
- **mTBI** = Minor (lower case letter M) traumatic brain injury.

A brain injury that is relatively mild and is commonly referred to as a concussion.

- **MTBI** = Major (upper case letter M) traumatic brain injury. A brain injury that is cause significant cellular damage and is often associated with intracranial bleeding.
- **Neuron** = A cell within the brain that carries or stores neurological information.
- **Neuroplasticity** = The process through which the brain develops new neuronal pathways to perform certain tasks.
- **Oleic Acid** = An omega-9 fatty acid that is very plentiful in olive oil. Oleic acid blocks the brain damage that can result from excessive omega-6 fatty acids and palmitic acid.
- **Omega-3 Fatty Acid** = These nutrients are unsaturated fatty acids and are important for normal metabolism. They are classified as an essential nutrient because humans are unable to synthesize omega-3 fatty acids and require them in their diet in order to remain healthy.
- **Omega-6 Fatty Acid** = These nutrients are a family of pro-inflammatory and anti-inflammatory polyunsaturated fatty acids. They are commonly found in plants and are classified as essential nutrients.
- **Omega-9 Fatty Acid** = These are unsaturated fatty acids and are not essential nutrients. Oleic acid found within olive oil is an example of an omega-9 fatty acid.
- **Palmitic Acid** = This nutrient is the most common saturated fatty acid found in animals, plants, and microorganisms. Excessive amounts in the diets of humans results in increase inflammation within the brain.
- **Phenotype** = The phenotype is the visible characteristic of how an animal, cell, or plant looks or behaves. (Genotype is the potential characteristic coded in the organism's DNA).
- **Prebiotic** = A form of fiber that induces the growth or activity of beneficial microorganisms (e.g., bacteria and

fungi). The most common example is in the gastrointestinal tract where the digestion of prebiotic fibers can alter the composition of organisms in the gut microbiome.

- **Probiotic** = Bacterial organisms that are ingested or added to foods, and are potentially beneficial to health.
- **Propionic Acid** = A small chain fatty acid produced by bacteria within the intestinal tract.
- **RifaGut**^{TM} = Another market brand name for rifaximin.
- **Rifaximin** = The generic term for the non-absorbable antibiotic sold under the brand name Xifaxan^{TM}, Rifagut^{TM}, Rifaximina^{TM} and SIBOFix^{TM}.
- **SIBO** = Small Intestine Bacterial Overgrowth. A specific form of bacterial overgrowth that is designated by a positive methane or hydrogen breath test or an abnormal quantification study from small intestinal aspirate.
- **SIBOFix**^{TM} = Another market brand name for rifaximin.
- **Synapse** = A portion of a neuron (or nerve cell) that permits the neuron to pass an electrical or chemical signal to another neuron.
- **The Nemechek Protocol**^{TM} = a medical treatment program invented by Dr. Patrick M. Nemechek, D.O. relating to methods for preventing, reducing, or reversing acute and/or chronic autonomic damage by the suppression of pro-inflammatory cytokines which is useful in treating a variety of diseases or conditions (Patent Pending).
- **Toxic Encephalopathy** = The medical state of a child whose brain has essentially been drugged with excessive propionic acid.
- **Traumatic Brain Injury, TBI** = The focal term for a physical injury to the head and results in symptoms lasting more than 24 hours. See mTBI and MTBI.
- **Vagus Nerve** = The 10th cranial nerve of the human body

that carries the signals in the parasympathetic branch of the autonomic nervous system.

- **Vagus Nerve Stimulation, VNS** = This is a medical treatment that involves delivering electrical impulses to the Vagus nerve in the autonomic nervous system. Therapeutically VNS reduces inflammation throughout the brain and body and is capable of inducing neuroplasticity.
- **White Blood Cells (WBC)** = Cells of the immune system are often referred to as white blood cells or WBCs.
- **Xifaxan**^{TM} = This is the brand name of a time-released formulation of rifaximin sold within the United States.

INTRODUCTION

"I can explain the underlying cause of most diseases in just 13 words: The failure of our brains sets into motion the failure of our bodies."

— Dr. Patrick M. Nemechek, D.O.

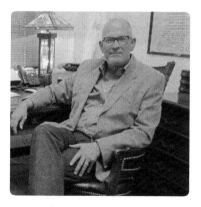

Dr. Patrick M. Nemechek, D.O. was born in Tucson, Arizona. He graduated with a B.S. in Microbiology from San Diego State University (1982), and obtained his Doctorate in Osteopathic Medicine from the University of Health Sciences, Kansas City, Missouri (1987).

Dr. Nemechek completed his training in internal medicine at UCLA School of Medicine (1990) where he had the distinguished honor of being named Chief Resident and later Clinical Instructor for the Department of Medicine at UCLA.

Dr. Nemechek's mentor at UCLA was Albert Einstein's nephew who encouraged him to go into the particularly complex field of HIV Medicine, which was the medical mystery of that time, where Dr. Nemechek would have the challenging freedom to save people's lives.

While at UCLA, Dr. Nemechek was recognized with the Robert S. Mosser Award for Excellence in Internal Medicine for his outstanding academic performance and instrumental role in starting UCLA's first HIV clinic at Kern Medical Center, Bakersfield, California.

In 1994, Dr. Nemechek moved to Kansas City, Missouri where he opened an HIV treatment and research facility named Nemechek Health Renewal.

It was at this point that Dr. Nemechek started work in earnest as a classically trained internal medicine "scientist-physician", entering the field of HIV when there was no diagnostic test, no treatment, and no answers.

Those early decades transformed Dr. Nemechek into an innovator who followed the latest research, looked at problems on a cellular and metabolic level, and became one of the first doctors to figure out ways to treat wasting syndrome as well as other HIV-related complex problems.

Dr. Nemechek's innovative approach to the complexities of HIV Disease garnered him honors such as being chosen as a "Site of Clinical Excellence" by Bristol Myers Squibb Company & KPMG Peat Marwick, being named one of the top HIV physicians in the U.S. by POZ magazine and receiving several nominations for the Small Business of the Year Award by the Greater Kansas City Chamber of Commerce.

During his 20 years in the Midwest, Dr. Nemechek authored or co-authored 72 scientific abstracts and publications, participated in 41 different clinical studies and in 1999 became a founding investigator for the HIV Research Network, a consortium of 18 different universities and HIV treatment facilities funded by the U.S. Department of Health and Human Services.

He has served on numerous editorial, professional and advisory boards as well as founding two non-profit HIV health advocacy organizations, the Bakersfield Aids Foundation and Fight Back KC.

By 2004, many of Dr. Nemechek's HIV patients were stable and leading normal lives but strangely they were starting to die of sudden cardiac events due to Cardiac Autonomic Neuropathy (CAN).

Dr. Nemechek set out to learn more about the lethal phenomena and in 2006 purchased new technology called spectral analysis that allowed him to tune into the communication signal between the heart and the brain, quantifying the balance and tone of the two branches of the autonomic nervous system.

Dr. Nemechek received additional training in autonomic testing and analysis at the Universidade De Lisboa, in Lisbon, Portugal, one of the top autonomic research facilities in the world.

Dr. Nemechek has now performed and analyzed thousands of autonomic patterns of damage. The more Dr. Nemechek learned about the field of Autonomic Medicine, the more he realized that it is the failure of the brain that sets into motion the failure of the body.

With his extensive research experience and expertise in metabolism, immunology, and the autonomic nervous system, Dr. Nemechek returned to his home state of Arizona in 2010 with his wife Jean and opened Nemechek Consultative Medicine, an Internal Medicine and Autonomic Medicine practice.

Jean Nemechek is uniquely qualified to run the business and co-author with Dr. Nemechek as she graduated with a B.A. in Communications and a B.S. in Journalism from the University of Kansas (1988, 1989) and a Juris Doctorate from Washburn School of Law (1993).

After relocating back home to Arizona, Dr. Nemechek was once again treating children and adults of all ages for routine matters. He was shocked at how incredibly

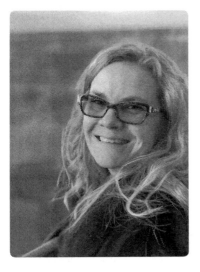

sick the general population had become in just a few decades. The disease continuum had moved up about 40 years it seemed, and diseases that had once struck only the elderly were routinely occurring in middle age or early adulthood.

Dr. Nemechek could recall when he was a medical student and his instructor called him into an exam room to see a person in their 50's who had diabetes. It was unheard of in those days to have someone "so young" with type II diabetes. Tragically that disease is now quite commonplace in middle age as we have become collectively sick and old at an accelerated pace.

Dr. Nemechek realized that many of his routine patients were suffering from the early stages of disease and autonomic dysfunction (heartburn, headaches, fatigue), small intestine bacterial overgrowths – SIBO (intestinal distress, food intolerances), and their children were increasingly experiencing the symptoms arising from autonomic dysfunction and SIBO (anxiety, ADD, autism, and digestive and intestinal issues).

And then is when Dr. Nemechek began, once again, to make history. He knew he had to change the practice of modern medicine back to the goals of healing the patient and reversing disease. Dr. Nemechek began to approach his regular patients with same the investigative research angle that he once did with HIV, he pushed beyond the disease labels to understand and resolve the underlying problem.

Dr. Nemechek started using all available scientific and medical tools to induce the nervous system and organs to repair themselves by normalizing inflammation control mechanisms, inducing natural stem cell production, and reactivating innate restorative mechanisms.

Starting in 2010, Dr. Nemechek embarked on an extraordinary path that involved altering and improving intestinal bacteria and reducing pro-inflammatory cytokines within the central nervous system, and witnessed unprecedented recovery in all five stages of autonomic dysfunction without long term medication. This is unheard of in our time.

As the years passed Dr. Nemechek also began working with various current and former professional athletes whose brain symptoms resolved (Autonomic Advantage™ Brain Injury Recovery Program), began offering expert opinions on Autonomic Medicine in the United States Court of Federal Claims, and he began incorporating bioelectric medicine, specifically electromodulation of the Vagus nerve, with his patients.

Dr. Nemechek found the key to treatment and reversal of many of the common diseases affecting people today is reversing dysfunction of the autonomic nervous system in combination with the renewal of stem cell production and neurogenesis through the reduction of metabolic inflammation.

Because of his efforts and career experiences, Dr. Nemechek invented an effective program to prevent, reduce, or reverse autonomic nervous system damage through a combination of natural neurochemical supplements, short term prescription medications, dietary restrictions, and neuromodulation of the Vagus nerve.

Dr. Nemechek's treatment approach is extremely effective in the recovery of autonomic function from a variety of neuroinflammatory conditions including traumatic brain injury, concussion, chronic traumatic encephalopathy (CTE), post-concussion syndrome (PCS), Alzheimer's disease, Parkinson's disease, essential tremor, post-traumatic stress disorder (PTSD), chronic depression, treatment resistant epilepsy, autism, developmental delay, Asperger's syndrome, and sensory and motor disorders.

In 2016, Dr. Nemechek filed a patent application to protect his groundbreaking formula that is now known as "The Nemechek Protocol™" or The Nemechek Protocol for Autonomic Recovery (Patent Pending).

In response to his unique expertise in clinical autonomics and the development of The Nemechek Protocol™ for Autonomic Recovery (Patent Pending), the practice was renamed (dba) Nemechek Autonomic Medicine in 2017.

This book explains the main tools used by Dr. Nemechek in his work with autistic and developmental delay patients in his medical practice using certain parts of The Nemechek Protocol™. His approach with these patients is now also commonly referred to as "The Nemechek Protocol™ for Autism", and it has spread throughout the world.

SETTING THE STAGE FOR AUTISM

BACTERIAL OVERGROWTH, PRIMED-MICROGLIA, AND INFLAMMATION

There is growing scientific evidence that an imbalance of intestinal bacteria along with excessive inflammation within the brain are responsible for the features associated with autism as well as ADD/ADHD, mood disorders, and developmental delay in children.

NORMAL BRAIN DEVELOPMENT

The Nemechek Protocol™ may help many of those childhood issues because they all have similar origins, specifically an overgrowth of intestinal bacteria and multiple mechanisms that fuel inflammation.

Normal brain development requires a healthy environment for the brain to develop fully and quickly. A child is born with approximately 100 billion neurons and they must trim these down to 50 billion neurons by the time they are 18 years old.

Failure to trim the neurons fast enough may lead to developmental issues. If the failure to trim is mild and the neurons simply are not being trimmed fast enough, we often refer to this as developmental delay.

If the neuronal trimming process has severely slowed or even stopped completely, the child may be classified as having mental retardation.

The common cause of altered neuronal pruning is from impaired functioning of a specialized central nervous system white blood cell known as microglia.

Microglia are often referred to as the 'master gardener' because one of their primary roles is to tend to the neurons that branch throughout the brain like the branches of plants throughout a garden.

Microglia tend to the neuron branches by either pruning them (getting rid of) or by protecting and repairing them.

The development and distribution of neurons is felt to be somewhat random as the child's brain is having to discover a connection between bodily movements and brain function.

The development process involves forming the pathways that will allow your child to track your face with their eyes, or roll over in the crib. These behaviors occur only when the child's brain finds the neurons that connect the thought (follow mother's face) to the action (move my eyes and head).

Microglia sense these neuronal pathways are important and start nurturing and protecting them. If other neurons are not being used in any meaningful way, they will eventually be trimmed away as excess.

The process of pruning away the excessive neurons is necessary for the brain to survive. Neurons consume large amounts of energy. It is inefficient for the human body to spend energy on pathways that are not important for survival.

At the time of birth the brain consumes nearly 85% of all oxygen and calories whereas it is "pruned down" to a mass by 18 years of age that only consumes 20%. From an evolutionary viewpoint, this is a much more manageable percentage.

The neuronal pruning process continues throughout the child's life as they learn to crawl, stand upright, talk, walk, run, read, calculate, and mature into young adults.

The microglia not only trim and maintain the normal sequence of maturation, they also help repair the brain injuries that can occur from physical (concussion and sub-concussive injuries), emotional (bullying, intense fear), and inflammatory (surgery, fractures, vaccinations) traumas.

Unfortunately, microglia function can be altered by the leakage of lipopolysaccharide (LPS), a fragment of bacterial cell membranes that is leaked into the blood stream when bacterial overgrowth of the small intestine occurs.

The microglia altered by LPS are referred to as primed microglia.

MICROGLIA AND ABNORMAL BRAIN DEVELOPMENT

In the womb, a child's intestinal tract contains no bacteria. It is only after a child is born that a child's intestinal tract becomes colonized with their mother's blend of bacteria.

Regardless whether the birth is vaginal or by caesarian section, the child's intestinal bacterial blend matches the bacterial blend of the mother. If the mother's bacterial blend is off a bit then the child's bacterial blend is off a bit as well.

But the bacterial issue is not just a mother-child issue, both parents contribute in different ways.

Which bacteria will overgrow, or what those bacteria might do once they overgrow, can be determined by the genes contributed by the mother or the father.

It is a complex combination of the mother's bacterial blend that may malfunction according to the father's genetic instructions.

Many, if not most individuals, have abnormal blends of intestinal bacteria to some degree. If the child's newly colonized intestinal bacterial is out of balance, bacterial overgrowth (SIBO) may occur shortly after birth.

And depending on the severity of the bacterial overgrowth, the impairment of microglial pruning may begin shortly after birth.

In other children, their bacterial blend may only be mildly imbalanced and incapable of triggering impairment of the microglia pruning process.

Their bacterial blend may require an additional push into full bacterial imbalance from a round of antibiotics, antacids, surgery, or a vaccination.

A SIMPLE DESCRIPTION OF BACTERIAL OVERGROWTH

Bacterial overgrowth is a condition where the child's own bacteria that should only reside at the bottom of their colon have replicated and migrated up to the child's small intestine.

This is a massive disruption in the normally balanced intestinal bacterial system. Bacteria from the colon are very different from the bacteria that live in the small intestine.

The two types of bacteria are so different that I explain to my patients that one type is like birds (the normal residents of the small intestine) and the other type is like fish (the normal residents of the colon).

The acidity of their respective environments, and the motility of the intestinal tract, seem to be the main reasons that these two types of bacteria remain separated.

The small intestine is a relatively acidic environment whereas the colon (large intestine) is much more alkaline.

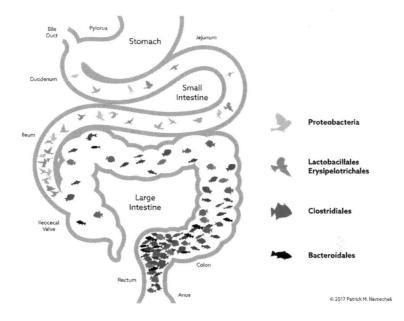

Normal Intestinal Bacterial Balance

Furthermore, there is a very large difference in the concentration of the bacteria. For every individual "bird" bacterium in the upper small intestine, there is normally a hundred million "fish" bacteria living in the lowest portion of the colon. That is an enormous difference.

Bacterial overgrowth occurs when the "fish" bacteria migrate up into the small intestinal tract and start living up with the "birds". Everyone understands that fish should not be living up with birds.

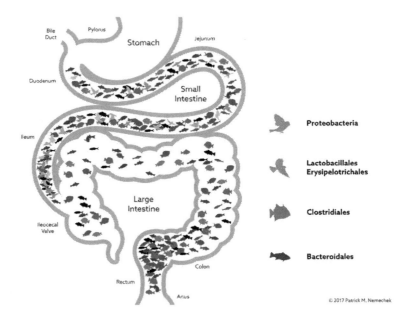

Bacterial Overgrowth of the Small Intestine

After they have migrated into the small intestine, colonic bacteria can create inflammation, influence cell behavior, produce acid, emit toxins and gases, get excited or react to different foods (tomatoes, bananas, milk, citrus, etc.), cause skin disruptions (eczema, hives, rashes), and send signals to the brain through the autonomic nervous system that disrupts brain, body, and cell function.

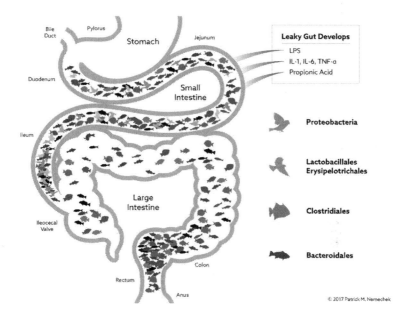

When bacterial overgrowth occurs fragments of bacteria cell membrane called lipopolysaccharide (LPS) leak into the blood stream and flow into the brain where the LPS alters the function of a special white blood cell known as microglia.

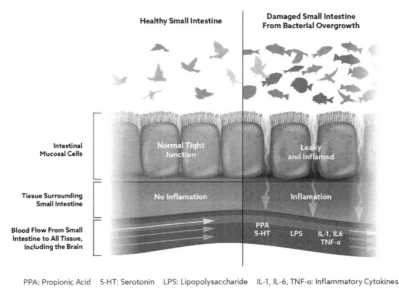

PPA: Propionic Acid   S-HT: Serotonin   LPS: Lipopolysaccharide   IL-1, IL-6, TNF-α: Inflammatory Cytokines

© 2017 Patrick M. Nemechek

We call these altered microglia "primed microglia" and their function changes from a helpful cell that repairs damaged neurons into an unhealthy cell that prevents normal development.

Whether bacterial overgrowth and LPS happen at the time of birth or happens later as the child is growing up, whenever the LPS leakage begins in earnest is when both improper neuronal pruning and the impairment of brain development begins.

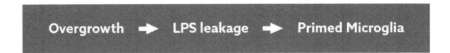

Adding to the impairment is a recent trend that we have seen in the last few decades which is the inability to fully repair the brain after common injuries that occur to children.

The common childhood injuries to which I refer are what used to be normal and insignificant falls and bumps to the head that all children experience as they crawl, walk, play, interact with siblings, and explore their environment.

There is often a crying child at the family reunion or at the park because they hit their head while playing. This is a normal type of injury that children used to fully recover from automatically.

Children would cry for a while, be comforted, calm down, and then they would be fine. We understand now that those simple head injuries more than likely cause minor brain damage that would fully be repaired with healthy microglia.

Unfortunately, the same minor injury is not fully repaired by the primed microglia that inhabit the brain of a child who has bacterial overgrowth.

The bacterial overgrowth of their small intestine interferes with the child's brain repair after a bump or fall because the microglia are no longer in a repair mode, instead the primed microglia have switched into a damage-causing mode.

Bacterial Overgrowth and Microglia Recap:

- Helpful, normal microglia help us develop normally during childhood.
- Colonic bacteria (fish) are migrating too high into the small intestine (birds).
- Bacterial overgrowth = when colonic bacteria (fish) are living up with the small intestine bacteria (birds).
- Bacterial overgrowth causes LPS leakage, which changes cell function to "Primed Microglia"
- Primed microglia are no longer helpful, primed microglia are harmful.
- Primed microglia do not perform normal neuron pruning or repair brain injuries.

PRIMED MICROGLIA MAGNIFY DAMAGE AND LIMIT RECOVERY

Primed microglia will also worsen the degree of damage caused by the injury and prevent stem cells and other repair mechanisms from fully repairing the brain damage that would have fully recovered in an otherwise healthy brain with normal functioning microglia.

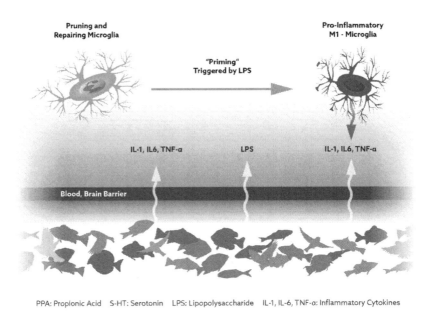

Pruning and Repairing Microglia

"Priming" Triggered by LPS

Pro-Inflammatory M1 - Microglia

IL-1, IL6, TNF-α   LPS   IL-1, IL6, TNF-α

Blood, Brain Barrier

PPA: Propionic Acid   S-HT: Serotonin   LPS: Lipopolysaccharide   IL-1, IL-6, TNF-α: Inflammatory Cytokines

© 2017 Patrick M. Nemechek

The impairment of microglia may also be responsible for the abnormal white matter structure within the brain that seems to be associated with sensory perception disorders.

More damage and less recovery are the hallmark features of a pathological process called cumulative brain injury or CBI.

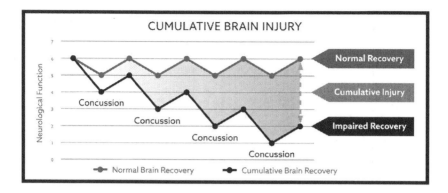

Cumulative brain injury from primed microglia is occurring in an epidemic fashion throughout the population, and is the predominant feature behind the well-publicized problems of professional football players contracting chronic traumatic encephalopathy (CTE).

Cumulative brain injury develops not only from physical injuries but can occur from emotional and inflammatory (surgery, fractures, vaccines) injuries as well.

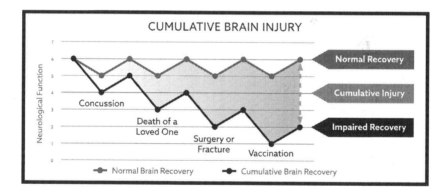

In addition to primed microglia not pruning correctly and causing varying degrees of developmental delay, the cumulative brain injury effect from primed microglia is also allowing small brain injuries to stack upon previously unresolved brain injuries.

This cumulative damage results in conditions such as attention deficit disorder (ADD), hyperactivity, headaches, anxiety, and chronic depression.

Primed Microglia ➡	Developmental Delay + Cumulative Brain Injury

If it is bad enough, the process of bacterial overgrowth will trigger developmental delay which may be mild or severe. In addition to this developmental delay, there may also be other conditions such as ADD, ADHD, fidgety movements, toe-walking, headaches, and anxiety that are from the child's cumulative brain injury.

The increase of inflammation within the central nervous system also lowers the seizure threshold and increases both the likelihood and the frequency of seizures. This effect is seen in its most benign form, which are called febrile seizures.

Increased Inflammation ➡ Increased Chance of Seizure

A febrile seizure is a minor and harmless seizure in small children that only lasts a few minutes and occurs when the child is running a temperature. This is an "out of the blue" event in an otherwise healthy child.

In this situation, the child develops an inflammatory response and a fever after contracting a common viral infection. The inflammation then lowers the seizure threshold causing the child to have a seizure.

These seizures do not return unless the fever and inflammatory reaction occur again. Fortunately, children grow out of this pattern once their nervous system matures further.

Bacterial overgrowth, LPS leakage, primed microglia, cumulative brain injury, and increased inflammation have now set the stage in the child and all it takes is one more pathological twist and autism occurs.

The feature that turns a child with developmental delay, ADD, headaches, and anxiety into a child who develops autism is the production of a short chain fatty acid called propionic acid.

2

SLIPPING INTO AUTISM

THE SEDATING EFFECT OF PROPIONIC ACID

There are thousands of different bacterial species within the colon that can potentially flux up into the small intestine and begin growing in excess.

Some of these bacteria come from the clostridium family, and when there is bacterial overgrowth they are given the opportunity to grown out of control and they can produce large amounts of propionic acid.

Propionic acid acts like a drug when there is enough in the body. When propionic acid levels rise in the brains of animals they begin behaving strangely as if intoxicated by a medication.

The same effect will happen with children when their intestinal tract is overgrown with enough propionic acid-producing bacteria. The stuporous state from propionic acid may occur in some children shortly after birth.

Other children may begin to hit their normal milestones and it is only after a course of antibiotics, a surgical procedure, a strong antacid, or a vaccination that their intestinal bacteria spin further out of control with the result being a spike in propionic acid production.

When this occurs, the parents see a sudden shift in the child's demeanor and behavior.

A child that might have only been showing some hints of developmental issues (e.g., not speaking or crawling as early as their sibling) suddenly ceases interacting with their environment. They quit noticing people and may stop speaking altogether.

These children have just been drugged with propionic acid because some external factor worsened the degree of their bacterial overgrowth and shifted it from a bacterial blend with the potential to produce propionic acid into one that is now producing large amounts of propionic acid.

The child is essentially being drugged with propionic acid and this medical state is referred to as a toxic encephalopathy.

The transition into autism begins whenever the propionic acid production levels are high enough to saturate the brain of the child and have begun their sedating effect on the child's behavior.

The timing of that increase of propionic acid explains why many parents report they observed their child change before their eyes while other parents report their child demonstrated autistic and other developmental features since birth.

Although a newborn child adopts their mother's intestinal bacterial blend at birth, many other factors are often involved for the child to slip into autism.

Those other factors influencing the child's bacterial blend could include a stay in the neonatal intensive care unit (NICU), a surgical procedure to repair a hole in the heart or pyloric stenosis, or the mother requiring IV antibiotics just prior to delivery to prevent group B Strep (GBS) from infecting the child (GBS infection can cause miscarriage, stillbirth, or death after birth).

A child's father can contribute to the child's risk of developing autism by contributing genes that (1) may favor the overgrowth of the propionic-producing clostridium bacteria, or (2) lead to microglia that are more sensitive to the priming effects of LPS.

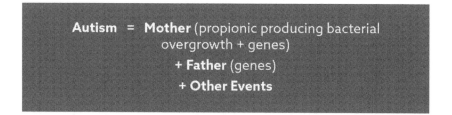

The difference between a child with developmental issues and ADD, when compared to a child with autism, developmental issues and ADD, is the production of large quantities of propionic acid.

And the difference between both of those examples when compared to a child with no evidence of autism, developmental delay, or any effects of cumulative brain injury (ADD, anxiety, or headaches), is the health of the microglia within the child's brain.

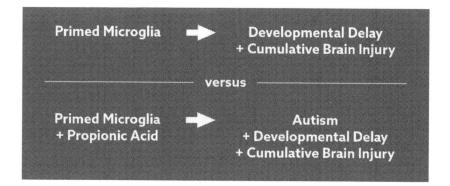

Once the bacterial overgrowth is reversed and propionic acid levels decline, and the children are released from the toxic, stuporous prison they have been trapped in. I refer to this as "the awakening period" in my patients.

During the awakening period, the child may become more energetic and alert. This awakening may manifest as being more observant and aware of their environment, more interactive, and even more calm.

On the other hand, some children in the awakening period will demonstrate the true extent of their underlying developmental issues, autonomic nervous system dysfunction, and their cumulative brain injury.

These awakened children may seem more anxious, engage in more stimulating behavior, act more anxious or aggressive, and sleep less. This is not a worsening of their autism as many fear, instead this is a child who is now fully alert without the sedating effects of propionic acid.

Fortunately, the brain has a remarkable capacity to begin trimming neurons and catching up developmentally, as well as repairing the underlying cumulative damage from past injuries.

I often say the process of catching up developmentally and repairing underlying brain injury is like watching your hair grow, it is a slow but steady process.

Day by day invisible recovery occurs, but before you know it a new behavior or a milestone is gained.

I remind my patient's families that this is a long term brain repair process. The gains we have seen on The Nemechek Protocol™ are unparalleled; we are in completely uncharted territory because the scope of this recovery has proven many theories about the impossibility of neurological recovery completely wrong.

In the future, I believe bacterial overgrowth may be found to be responsible for the production of a variety of other toxic encephalopathies.

Several examples of what I have seen in my patients is their recovery from stuttering, intense anxiety, insomnia, migraine headaches, dyslexia, tics, and chronic hiccups within a few weeks after restoring intestinal balance.

Each of these disorders could potentially be triggered by an unusual chemical produced by a unique strain of overgrown bacteria.

INFLAMMATION AND GENETIC ABNORMALITIES

It is quite clear that autism and other pervasive developmental disorders are increasing in incidence and the wide variety of genetic mutations in certain cases have direct impact on the features of these disorders.

Autism is associated with a wide variety of genetic mutations that form the basis of autism, with hundreds of genes providing varying degrees of risk.

Some of these genes are also being understood to be risk factors for other developmental disorders.

While some autism genes have an obvious functional significance (SHANKs, neuroligins, and neurexins, fragile x syndrome, mental retardation-associated proteins), many autism genes do not present a clear mechanism of dysfunction. The clinical significance of these non-associated genes has yet to be determined.

When speaking of the impact of genetics concerning any medical disorder that is increasing in frequency, one needs to try to understand whether these genes are new within in the affected individual (such as can happen with radiation exposure or drug exposure during pregnancy) or whether the genes were pre-existing, but dormant, in the donor parent from whom they were passed.

Inflammation may play a role in both new or dormant genes. Elevated levels of pro-inflammatory cytokines are capable of activating genes that have laid dormant in preceding generations.

Systemic inflammation can also impair the ability of stem cells to mature properly and cause DNA to be miscopied (genetic 'typos') especially when the child is developing within the womb.

In either scenario, it is more than likely that prior generations did not have as high of a prevalence of autism as we do today because they lived in an environment that produced much less inflammation within their bodies.

Prior to birth, inflammatory cytokines capable of causing mutations or activating pre-existent genes are produced within the mother's body, and they can influence the development or activation of the unborn child's cellular DNA.

Sources of inflammation within pregnant women and newborn children includes:

1. Primed CNS (Central Nervous System) Microglia from Bacterial Overgrowth
2. Deficient Dietary Omega-3 Fatty Acid Intake
3. Excess Dietary Omega-6 Fatty Acids Intake
4. Damage to the Autonomic Nervous System and the Vagus Inflammatory Reflex
5. Excessive Ingestion of Saturated Fatty Acids
6. Excessive Ingestion of Processed Carbohydrates
7. Ingestion of Advanced Glycation End Products (AGEs)
8. First or Second-Hand Tobacco Exposure
9. Autoimmune Disorders
10. Probiotic Use

This is an extensive list of sources of metabolic inflammation but numbers 1 - 4 are the most common factors that seem to affect the health of the patients, both young and old, that I see in my practice.

Reduction of those sources of inflammation within both children and pregnant mothers may serve two distinct purposes regarding the development of autism.

In pregnant mothers, less systemic inflammation will allow neuronal stem cells to develop correctly and more fully, and would therefore lessen the likelihood of genetic mutations being activated or created.

In children, less systemic inflammation will allow microglia and cellular repair mechanisms to function more normally and effectively, thereby promoting neuronal pruning and a normal pace of development.

Significant reductions of inflammation within the child may also allow abnormally activated genes to be switched off and cease causing harm to the individual.

3
———

THE INFLAMMATORY-NEUROTOXIC SPECTRUM

Historically, when scientists have tried to understand certain abnormal behaviors in individuals, they will group patients together under a certain heading based on their particular observed abnormal behavior.

Their approach is not much different than trying to figure out a 1,000-piece jigsaw puzzle.

Most of us will begin to organize the puzzle pieces according to certain characteristics such as a particular color, patterns, or pieces than encompass the middle or the flat edge of the puzzle.

Doing this helps us to make sense of a wide variety of seemingly unrelated pieces.

An example of the jigsaw puzzle approach is based on observed, abnormal emotional behavior under terms such as depression, anxiety, schizophrenia, psychosis, and personality disorders.

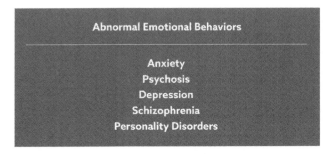

Another grouping based on observed characteristics is the developmental disorders that affect children.

DEVELOPMENTAL DIAGNOSES ARE BASED ON OBSERVED BEHAVIORS

The developmental jigsaw puzzle consists of observed autism spectrum disorders (autism, Asperger syndrome, or Pervasive Developmental Disorder-Not Otherwise Specified), pervasive developmental disorders (delays in the development of multiple basic functions), specific developmental disorders (delays in only a specific area), and other neurodevelopmental disorders such as traumatic brain injury (TBI), and attention deficit disorders (ADD, ADHD).

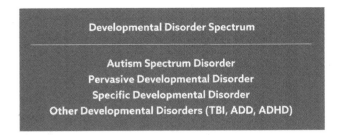

This system works well in the respect that a wide variety of research has shown that this particular treatment approach may help one aspect developmental disorder more than another.

It also serves as a platform to help manage distribution of

supportive resources (therapists, medical care, school assistance, etc.) more efficiently.

The problem is that this observed organizational approach is not useful when trying to understand the underlying cause of many developmental disorders of children.

A COMMON PATHOLOGICAL PROCESS FOR MANY DEVELOPMENTAL DISORDERS

A broad range of studies are outlining a process in which the combination of abnormal microglia (a white blood cell) functioning and elevated levels of pro-inflammatory cytokines within the central nervous system play a significant role in the development of a wide range of neurological disorders in both adults and children.

In adults, the abnormal activation of microglia and elevated cytokines are associated with an increased risk of developing Alzheimer's disease, Parkinson's disease, amyotrophic lateral sclerosis (ALS), macular degeneration, treatment-resistant epilepsy, chronic depression and post-traumatic stress disorder, post-concussion syndrome, as well as chronic traumatic encephalopathy (CTE) in athletes.

In children, this same pathological process is associated with impaired development of fundamental brain architecture, neuron and synaptic pruning (developmental delay), and the incomplete recovery from physical, emotional, and inflammatory brain trauma (cumulative brain injury).

Therefore, in order to clearly understand how a single approach can positively affect so many seemingly different forms of childhood developmental issues, the approach needs to be viewed from the common pathway of microglia activation and pro-inflammatory cytokines.

I refer to this viewpoint as the inflammatory-neurotoxic spectrum of developmental disorders.

THE INFLAMMATORY-NEUROTOXIC SPECTRUM OF DEVELOPMENTAL DISORDERS

Instead of viewing developmental disorders from the perspective of the child's observed behavior, a clearer picture of the disease process is gained by viewing the disease process from a cellular pathological process.

The variety of abnormal behavioral patterns is a reflection of the variety of different areas of the brain that are not functioning correctly. The concept is no different than observing the variety of manners in which a stroke may affect an adult.

Some adults with a stroke may have paralysis of both their right arm and leg, others may have weakness in the left arm and are unable to speak or swallow, while others may simply begin to manifest dementia without any impairment of their limbs at all.

Each of these patterns of altered neurological function represent a different area of the brain that is affected. The same holds true for children with developmental disorders.

The wide variation of speech, sensory, motor, cognition, and emotional difficulties a child may experience simply represents the summation of different areas of their brain not working correctly.

The chronic brain dysfunction in children with developmental disorders can occur through three different processes which are:

1. Unrepaired brain trauma (cumulative brain injury),
2. A slow rate or abnormal process of neuronal pruning (developmental delay)
3. Toxic encephalopathy (propionic acid toxicity).

A small proportion of children may also be negatively affected by genetic mutations.

All of these pathological processes are worsened with an increase in systemic and central nervous system inflammation that comes from a variety of sources, but it is the bacterial overgrowth from the intestinal tract that seems to contribute the most to this inflammation.

Bacterial overgrowth also contributes to the production of propionic acid that has a toxic effect on brain function in a fashion similar to a sedative such as Valium® (diazepam) or a hallucinogen such as LSD (lysergic acid diethylamide).

THE CASCADING EFFECT OF INFLAMMATION AND BACTERIAL OVERGROWTH

The inflammatory spectrum starts with a mild degree of inflammation.

The inflammation first impairs the ability of the brain to fully repair from the common physical, emotional, and inflammatory brain injuries that can occur during childhood.

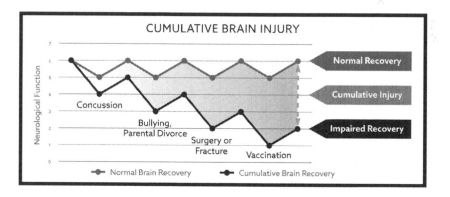

The residual damage accumulates over time in a process called cumulative brain injury and can result in common developmental problems such as attention deficit disorder (ADD), hyperactivity, increased hunger or thirst, chronic depression, aggression, or generalized anxiety.

As the inflammation builds further, the natural process of neuronal and synaptic pruning in a child is negatively affected.

The child begins missing developmental milestones involved with speech, socialization, or play and is diagnosed with some form of developmental delay.

The slow rate of pruning of excessive neurons is a direct reflection of excessive inflammation within the central nervous system.

The sources of this growing tide of inflammation are varied. The primary source in most children comes from the bacterial over-growth within the intestinal tract.

Deficiencies of omega-3 fatty acid (fish, fish oil, nuts) intake combined with excessive exposure to inflammatory dietary omega-6 fatty acids (soy oil and other vegetable oils) are other major contributing factors.

The final stage in the inflammatory spectrum is a worsening of bacterial overgrowth to the degree that the neuronal pruning has slowed so much there is now developmental arrest, much more severe degrees of cumulative brain injury.

Added to this is the toxic effect of propionic acid triggering the unique behaviors associated with autism (loss of eye contact, decreased engagement with others, obsession with spinning objects, stimming, repetitive behaviors, etc.).

The Inflammatory-Neurotoxic Spectrum

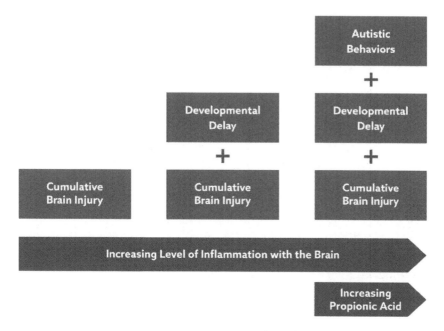

As the above graphic illustrates, any child diagnosed with even a single developmental disorder is at risk of also developing cumulative brain injury (CBI).

The cumulative brain injury may manifest as hyperactivity, increased hunger or thirst, aggression, anxiousness, extreme emotional sensitivity, or attention deficit disorder.

And as inflammation worsens and propionic acid levels increase within the brain, autistic behaviors begin to manifest.

The neuronal pruning may also worsen and can affect a wider range of brain regions leading to more pervasive pattern of developmental issues (PDD or PDD-NOS).

Worsening inflammation may cause or trigger underlying genetic mutations that lead to the most severe forms of autism with seizures and developmental arrest, and severe degrees of cumulative brain injury leading to extreme anxiety, aggression, cognitive impairment and a wide variety of autonomic nervous system dysfunction.

TARGETING TREATMENT FOR AUTISM AND DEVELOPMENTAL DISORDERS

Viewing the developmental disorders of childhood through the lens of inflammation and propionic acid toxicity helps to explain how such a simple treatment regimen as The Nemechek Protocol™ may affect so many seemingly different disorders.

The fact is that the underlying process that causes a large proportion of these disorders is one and the same. The childhood disorders differ only in respect to the area of the brain that is damaged and by what degree, along with whether or not the child experiences the additional toxic effect of propionic acid.

My model for autism is best understood as a theoretical model that is based on a wide variety of animal and human based research.

To be a definitive model, large scale, placebo-controlled human trials are needed but I know of no evidence that anyone is even considering conducting such a trial at the present time, especially for something as inexpensive and accessible as fish oil, olive oil, and inulin (or rifaximin).

One thing is for sure: my simple approach to inflammation and propionic acid suppression is having an unprecedented effect on many children around the world.

And that is proof enough that this model is correct to a substantial degree.

4

UNDERSTANDING HOW THE NEMECHEK PROTOCOL WORKS

AUTISM = PROPIONIC ACID + INFLAMMATION

The Nemechek Protocol™ helps a variety of childhood issues and disorders that surprisingly share the similar origins of an overgrowth of intestinal bacteria and multiple mechanisms that fuel inflammation.

Childhood developmental disorders (developmental delay, ADD, ADHD) and childhood mood disorders (anxiety, chronic depression, OCD) are primarily the consequence of excessive brain inflammation from intestinal bacteria.

Autism is the consequence of excessive brain inflammation in addition to a toxic encephalopathy from the overproduction of propionic acid from intestinal bacterial overgrowth.

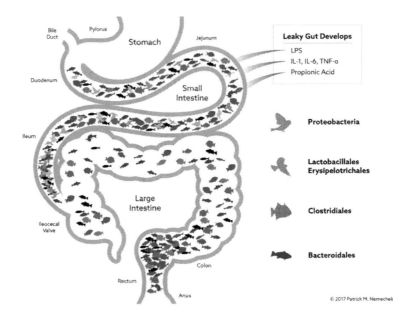

The propionic acid and inflammation contribute to the common features associated with autism as well as result in developmental delay or developmental arrest and cumulative brain injury (CBI) from unresolved brain trauma.

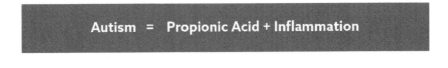

Autism = Propionic Acid + Inflammation

The excessive tissue/brain levels of propionic acid come from the intestinal tract and is produced by the abnormal presence of colon bacterial within the small intestine.

The inflammation is from excessive levels of pro-inflammatory cytokines within the brain. These cytokines are produced within the brain and throughout the body from a variety of sources. They are able to penetrate the blood brain barrier as well as freely flow into the brain via the paraventricular organs.

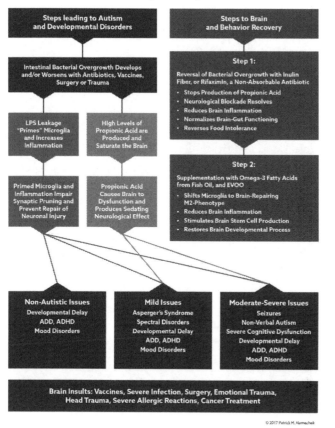

Autism and Other Childhood Developmental Disorders:
The Steps to Recovery

2-Step Process for The Nemechek Protocol

Therefore, my treatment of the core features of autism involves two general phases:

1. Reduction of Propionic Acid Levels Through the Reversal of Bacterial Overgrowth
2. Reduction of Pro-Inflammatory Cytokines Production from 3 - 4 Main Sources

In my patients who are children, it seems much less effort is required to reverse these processes and shift the body back into a healthier state than is required in my adult patients with similar issues.

The Nemechek Protocol™ is a long term brain recovery program, and it is measured in years. Therefore, when I say less effort is required with children than adults I do not mean less time, I mean they can have a better response without using pharmaceuticals.

It is my experience that most of my child patients respond to a consistent yet simple recipe of non-pharmaceutical fiber, inexpensive core nutrients, and a shift in dietary omega fatty acids.

Adult patients, however, often need short term pharmaceuticals and they do not respond as well to the non-pharmaceutical fiber.

GENERAL PHASE ONE

We are accustomed to thinking that our brains are in control over all of the things in our bodies. But the truth is that our intestinal tract can make chemicals and inflammation which impair brain function and development.

In this way, the intestinal tract's excessive propionic acid production is in control over the brain. This is why the first general phase of the Nemechek Protocol™ is focused on rebalancing the patient's intestinal tract.

Halting excessive propionic acid production from intestinal bacteria is achieved by re-balancing intestinal bacteria with either a prebiotic fiber called inulin (OTC) or with a non-absorbable antibiotic called rifaximin (RX).

Once excessive propionic acid production is reduced, cytokine production from intestinal bacterial translocation is also reduced.

The cumulative effect of treatment reverses the toxic effect of propionic acid as levels decline, and a reduction in inflammation triggers normal neuronal pruning and the improvement or reversal of even long-standing developmental delay.

GENERAL PHASE TWO

The second general phase involves a reduction in systemic (entire body) pro-inflammatory cytokine levels that prevent proper brain development or repair.

This involves attacking the most common sources of cytokine production in these children.

The four target sources of cytokines are:

1. Bacterial Translocation ('leaky gut') from Intestinal Overgrowth.
2. Abnormally-Activated ('primed') M1-Microglia within the Brain
3. Deficient Intake of Dietary Omega-3 Fatty Acids.
4. Excessive Intake of Dietary Omega-6 Fatty Acids.

REDUCING INFLAMMATORY CYTOKINES OVERVIEW:

The first target source of cytokine production overlaps with phase one, telling us just how important it is to address the intestinal overgrowth issue in children.

The reduction of bacterial overgrowth and excessive propionic acid with either the prebiotic inulin fiber (OTC) or the use of rifaximin (RX) also helps to reduce cytokine production from intestinal bacterial translocation.

The start of the healing chain of events lies in the intestinal tract to reduce bacterial overgrowth to stop excessive propionic acid, to then reduce cytokines, and to help reduce inflammation which allows the brain to begin to recover.

At this point, we focus our cytokine reduction efforts outside of the intestinal tract and into our diets and the rest of our body, in terms of different types of omega fatty acids that either help us or hurt us.

The foods we eat today are deficient in the omega-3 fatty acids that kept the brains and nervous systems in our ancestors strong, which is an important part of cytokine control.

There are three components of omega-3 fatty acids: DHA, EPA, and ALA. These components help our white blood cells function normally and control inflammation, and promote the lifelong production of stem cells throughout the body.

The deficient intake of all three components of dietary omega-3 fatty acids is satisfied by supplementation from fish oil (EPA and DHA) and plants (ALA).

While all three components of omega-3 fatty acids are necessary, the DHA component is our most effective tool against harmful microglia.

The suppression of the primed M1-microglia is obtained by the DHA component of omega-3 fatty acid found in fish oil. The other omega-3 fatty acids components (EPA and ALA) do not penetrate the brain nor do they suppress M1-microglia.

The next source of cytokine production is not what is missing in our diet, but an excessive amount of omega-6 fatty acids that have been added to our diets and cooking methods which compete with omega-3's and impair stem cell production.

There must be a reduction of excessive omega-6 fatty acids from cooking oils. The reduction in exposure from high concentration omega-6 fatty acid cooking and vegetables oils is also done by eliminating processed or prepared foods that contain these oils.

The trick is that most food labels do not list omega-6 oils. I instruct my patients to read ingredient lists and look for the most common things that contain omega-6 which are margarine, soybean oil, soy oil, grapeseed oil, safflower oil, and sunflower oil.

As my patients decrease omega-6 from cooking and vegetables oils, they also need to consume and cook with an omega-9 fatty acid to both heal from and block the harmful effects of omega-6.

This protection is found in oleic acid, an omega-9 fatty acid, which is found in domestic extra virgin olive oil.

If dietary changes and high doses of fish oil do not seem to achieve the desired cytokine reduction effect over time, I may consider the use of transcutaneous (on top of the skin) Vagus nerve stimulation for my patients.

The Vagus nerve is the 10th cranial nerve of the human body that carries the signals in the parasympathetic branch of the autonomic nervous system.

Vagus nerve stimulation is a safe, painless, bioelectric approach to aid in the reduction in central nervous system pro-inflammatory cytokine levels.

THE NEMECHEK PROTOCOL™ FOR AUTISM: AN OVERVIEW

The Nemechek Protocol™ for Autonomic Recovery (Patent Pending) is applicable to a variety of disease states in adults and children.

The Nemechek Protocol™ for Autism is just one part of that larger treatment program focused on brain and intestinal health, inflammation control, and improved autonomic nervous system function.

The Nemechek Protocol™ for Autism has four essential steps (1 - 4), and one optional step 5.

Many of my patients feel substantial recovery due to the reversal of autonomic nervous system dysfunction from steps 1 - 4.

1. Balance Intestinal Bacteria.
2. Shift M1-Microglia towards the Anti-Inflammatory M2-Microglia Phenotype.
3. Balance Omega-6 & Omega-3 Fatty Acids.

4. Reduction of Brain and Systemic Inflammation from Dietary Linoleic, Arachidonic, and Palmitic Acid.
5. Induction of Neuroplasticity.

Depending on my patient's health and response, optional step 5 may be added if warranted.

Now that you have an overview of the phases of intestinal rebalancing and cytokine control, and an introduction to The Nemechek Protocol™, I will explain how I use these tools in my patients to help reverse the core features of autism.

STEP 1: REBALANCING THE INTESTINAL TRACT

I t is estimated that most of us now have bacterial overgrowth to some degree.

Because a core feature of autism is the production of propionic acid from bacterial overgrowth, establishing control over bacterial overgrowth is the first essential, if not the critical, step of The Nemechek Protocol™.

Some children and adults with intestinal bacterial overgrowth will exhibit signs or symptoms of the overgrowth. Common symptoms of bacterial overgrowth include reflux or heartburn, food intolerances, constipation, anxiety, or eczema.

But it is not unusual for a child or an adult with bacterial overgrowth to not have any particular intestinal symptoms. Approximately 20% of adults with intestinal bacterial overgrowth have no obvious intestinal symptoms.

Although there may be no noticeable intestinal symptoms, bacterial overgrowth is still capable of producing toxic levels of propionic acid and preventing both neuronal pruning and brain injury repair through elevated brain inflammation and abnormal microglia function.

Because of those reasons, I believe all of my patients who are children with any aspect of autism or developmental delay issues need to address intestinal imbalance issues with one of the following options:

Preferred Method to Balance Intestinal Bacteria in Children 10 Years or Younger:

Inulin Prebiotic Fiber Supplementation
1/8 -1/4 teaspoon of inulin powder, 1-2 times per day.

Inulin is an over-the-counter (OTC) prebiotic fiber that comes from a variety of natural plant sources. Inulin derived from agave, chicory root, and Jerusalem artichoke are all acceptable forms of inulin. Inulin prebiotic powder is inexpensive and is sold by a variety of manufacturers.

My patients take 1/8 to 1/2 teaspoon of inulin powder, one to two times a day. The maximum inulin dose I use in older, larger children is 2 teaspoons per day.

Beyond the dose of 2 teaspoons a day, I have not witnessed any additional improvement in symptoms and it seems to cause discomfort in my patients from too much gas and bloating.

Inulin powder is odorless and tasteless. Inulin powder may be taken with or without food, it may be mixed with hot or cold solids, or it may be added to hot or cold liquids.

It has been my experience that the intestinal tract in some of my patients may go through some minor adjustments for a week or two after starting the inulin fiber.

These adjustments may include little intestinal issues such as constipation and bloating, but these things tend to straighten themselves out over time.

Inulin is the only prebiotic fiber that I use with my patients. Over the years I have tried different prebiotic and probiotic fibers in my office but none of them reduced bacterial overgrowth in a manner that allowed brain recovery to begin.

Inulin prebiotic fiber is a safe and natural plant fiber that is found in many foods we eat each day such as onions, artichokes, garlic, and in a wide variety of other vegetables.

Inulin increases the acidity of the small intestine which results in suppressed growth of the colonic bacteria within the small intestine. When the growth of the colonic bacteria is suppressed, propionic acid production is dramatically reduced.

Propionic acid is a chemical compound that our bodies naturally produce so it is not something that we can completely stop, but it is something that we may greatly reduce if it is made excessively by bacterial overgrowth.

Inulin fiber does not kill intestinal bacteria, instead it works like a fertilizer. Inulin fiber nourishes the healthy bacteria that rightfully should be living in the small intestine. The invading bacteria from the colon are not nourished by the inulin.

One very important point that I teach my patients is that prebiotic fibers are very different from probiotic bacteria.

Inulin is *not* a probiotic and inulin should *not* be used with a probiotic.

And all of my patients are instructed to immediately stop the use of all probiotics.

In an earlier chapter I explained how the bacteria in the small intestine are so different from the bacteria living down in the colon that you could think of one type of them as birds (small intestine bacteria) and the other type as fish (colon bacteria).

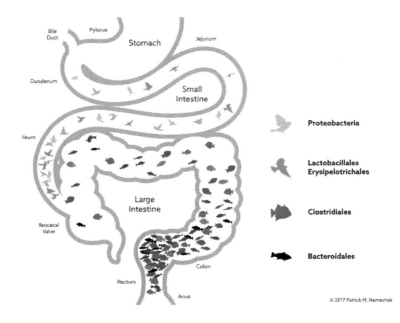

Normal Intestinal Bacterial Balance

Bacterial overgrowth is when your fish are living up with your birds, and their migration and replication creates approximately 10,000 to 100,000 times the normal number of bacteria within the small intestines.

This excessive number of bacteria overwhelm the protective barrier of the small intestine and results in bacterial translocation called "leaky gut".

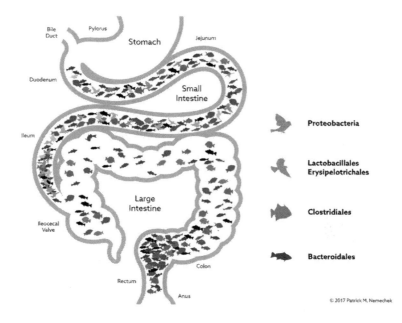

Unhealthy Bacterial Overgrowth

I tell my patients to think of inulin fiber as a healthy bacterial bird food for the small intestine: inulin feeds the birds (the good bacteria that should be there) but does not feed the fish (the invading bacteria).

Inulin powder also comes in the form of chewable gummies (including Fiber Choice®, Phillips' ® Fiber Good® Gummies). It has been my experience that two inulin gummies per day is enough to balance the intestinal tract in young children.

1/8 to 1/2 teaspoon of inulin powder, one to two times a day, or two inulin gummies a day, are the typical amounts my young patients consume.

I have also found that each child and their health needs may be different, and that bigger or older children with autism may require higher doses of inulin to control their bacterial overgrowth.

After starting my patient on daily inulin and fish oil, parents will ask how will they know whether this is the right amount of inulin and fish oil for their child. The treatment goals are:

Goal 1: The adequate reversal of bacterial overgrowth with inulin will lead to a drop in propionic acid and what I refer to as the awakening period in Chapter 6.

This is a period where a change in the patient occurs such as more eye contact, more alertness, more engagement, and possibly more stimming or insomnia.

Once a parent sees a change in my patient then the dose of inulin is adequate because the child has responded to that dose.

Goal 2: Improvements in neurological development will slowly move forward over the months. If there is improvement, then the parent knows my patient's dose of omega-3 fatty acids from fish oil is adequate.

If there is no significant improvement after two months then I will consider doubling the patient's omega-3 intake.

Pointers:

What type of inulin do I prefer? I prefer pure inulin powder for my patients. When buying powdered inulin, I avoid ones that also contain any probiotics or digestive enzymes because these ingredients can cause side effects of their own and may make some aspects of autism worse.

When might my patients first respond to treatment? Depending on the child's amount of underlying developmental delay, children may start making eye contact, allowing physical contact, or otherwise communicating and speaking within a few weeks to a few months.

Cases involving severe levels of developmental delay can take longer for speech or interaction to begin because the children appear to pick up where they had left off, wherever that may have been, from a developmental standpoint.

How long do my patients need to stay on inulin and the rest of The Nemechek Protocol™? Propionic acid control and brain recovery are long term processes.

There are some studies that indicate that developmental delay recovers at about a rate of two to three months for every calendar month that brain inflammation is lowered. This is fantastic motivation for consistent, persistent, propionic acid and inflammation control efforts in the years and decades ahead.

Have I seen intestinal symptoms change after starting inulin? Sometimes my patient's constipation or bloating seems to get worse after starting inulin. This is typically the result of underlying autonomic nervous system dysfunction that has slowed down the intestinal tract.

It has been my experience that these issues eventually resolve as other parts of The Nemechek Protocol™ improve autonomic function.

If those issues do not resolve or the child is too uncomfortable, I will generally recommend a non-fiber, non-digestive enzyme supplement such as magnesium (milk of magnesia) or MiraLAX® if constipation starts.

What if the inulin seems to worsen stemming? If there seems to be excessive stimming after starting the inulin, I'll recommend decreasing the inulin dose by an 1/8-1/4 a tsp per day and see if things improve. On rare occasions, increasing the inulin dose by that amounts may help as well.

Have I heard of cramping or mucous in stool? If my patient is experiencing cramping or mucous in stool, I first make sure they are still not getting any probiotics or digestive enzymes in any supplements or in their foods.

If this is not the case, I recommend stopping the inulin for a week and then restarting at a lower dose.

What if my patient cannot tolerate inulin? It may take several start-and-stop cycles to transition a child onto inulin fiber, and I prefer using this natural plant fiber with my patients.

But if I have a young patient who is unable to tolerate inulin over time then I may consider using a short course of the prescription rifaximin, the medicine that I use with older children.

What about other products for bacterial overgrowth? Inulin is the only fiber that that I use to rebalance or re-arrange bacterial overgrowth.

I do not use or recommend the use any other fibers, supplements, vitamins, minerals, herbs, or enzymes for bacterial overgrowth for my patients.

Do I test my patients for bacterial overgrowth, propionic acid, or types of bacteria in stools? No.

Warning:

My patients do not take probiotics during or after the use of inulin.

The reason why my patients are prohibited from taking probiotics during or after the use of inulin is once they are separating and rebalancing the birds and the fish back to their respective environments, the last thing I want them to do is to introduce brand new invaders (like lizards) for their birds to have to deal with.

Preferred Method to Balance Gut Bacteria, Children Older than 10 Years of Age:

Non-Absorbable Antibiotic
Rifaximin 550 mg twice daily for 10 days.

It has been my experience that children older than ten years of age tend not to get as complete of a recovery or as complete amount of control over their propionic acid toxicity from daily inulin supplementation.

The reasons for this are unclear and it may simply be related to a greater bacterial burden or more imbalance with bacteria within the biofilm layer.

If inulin fiber has been ineffective over time, or the older patient's symptoms are too severe, I will consider the use of one course of rifaximin (brand name Xifaxan®) 550 mg two times daily for 10 days to reduce the excessive colonic bacteria from the small intestine in my patients.

This is a prescription drug that must be prescribed and supervised by a physician. This pharmaceutical treatment may need to be periodically repeated by a child's physician as they see fit, as relapses of bacterial overgrowth are possible.

It is important to understand that treatment with inulin or rifaximin alone will not repair a child's brain. The key features of autism involve both brain inflammation and intestinal overgrowth issues that require long term brain inflammation and intestinal overgrowth reduction efforts.

Reducing propionic acid toxicity is just one of four basic parts in The Nemechek Protocol™ for Autism. I emphasize to my patient's parents that this is a four-part program, this is not an a la carte list for them to pick and choose from.

The patients in my office who are doing The Nemechek Protocol™ must simultaneously address brain inflammation and autonomic dysfunction with sufficient omega-3 fatty acids and omega-9 fatty acids, and the reduction of dietary omega-6 fatty acids.

After my patient completes their 10-day course of rifaximin and continues forward on their fish oil, parents will ask how will they know whether this was the right amount of rifaximin and fish oil for their child. The treatment goals are:

Goal 1: The adequate reversal of bacterial overgrowth with one course (10 days) of rifaximin will lead to a drop in propionic acid and what I refer to as the awakening period in Chapter 6.

This is a period where a change in the patient occurs such as more eye contact, more alertness, more engagement, and possibly more stimming or insomnia.

Once a parent sees a change in my patient then that dose was adequate because the child has responded to that dose.

Goal 2: Improvements in neurological development will slowly move forward over the months. If there is improvement, then the parent knows my patient's dose of omega-3 fatty acids from fish oil is adequate.

If there is no significant improvement after two months then I will consider doubling the patient's omega-3 intake.

Monitoring:

In some cases, bacterial overgrowth may be detected with a hydrogen and/or methane breath test. Treatment with rifaximin often results in the reversal of the findings on the breath test.

But from a practical stand point I quit using the breath test a long time ago with my patients because the breath test results did not help me identify whether or not someone needed treatment for bacterial overgrowth.

Many of my patients would improve despite having a test that was negative for bacterial overgrowth.

So instead I make very precise notes about the clinical improvements of intestinal, musculoskeletal, and neurological improvements in my patients that occurred within the first months after treatment.

I then use these changes to monitor if bacterial overgrowth relapses because the relapse will often result in the return of many of the same symptoms that resolved originally on inulin or rifaximin.

Pointers:

Follow-up use of inulin after rifaximin is sometimes used if intestinal symptoms such as diarrhea, post meal stool urgency, or food intolerance are still present. If inulin does not make any significant difference as a follow-up therapy, I stop using it in my patients.

I never add probiotics to my patient's treatment program after rebalancing intestinal overgrowth with rifaximin because the addition of probiotics can easily make things worse for the patient even if they helped prior to the use of rifaximin.

I have seen the addition of unknown strains of foreign bacteria (probiotics) increase my patient's inflammation, intestinal distress, depression, and other psychological symptoms.

Warning:

Rifaximin is a prescription medication and it should only be administered and supervised by a pediatrician, family physician, or a gastroenterologist.

With the exception of using inulin for continued diarrhea, etc., the continued use of prebiotics such as inulin, probiotics, or digestive enzymes after taking rifaximin is generally not recommended because they may cause a worsening of symptoms after intestinal bacterial re-balancing is achieved.

6

STEP 2-4: REDUCTION OF BRAIN INFLAMMATION

In the previous chapter I explained how cytokines from bacterial translocation are reduced with the rebalancing of intestinal bacteria in step 1 with inulin or rifaximin. In this chapter I will explain the next steps of Nemechek Protocol™ steps 2 through 4, and optional steps 5 and 6:

1. Balance Intestinal Bacteria.
2. Shift M1-Microglia towards the Anti-Inflammatory M2-Microglia Phenotype.
3. Balance Omega-6 to Omega-3 Fatty Acids.
4. Reduction of Brain and Systemic Inflammation from Dietary Linoleic, Arachidonic, and Palmitic Acids.
5. Induction of Neuroplasticity.

STEP 2. SHIFTING M1-MICROGLIA TO THE ANTI-INFLAMMATORY M2-PHENOTYPE

Steps 2 - 4 involves reducing cytokines from M1-microglia and the imbalance of omega-3 and omega-6 fatty acids.

Equally important as treating bacterial overgrowth are the next three essential steps of shifting microglia cells back to an anti-inflammatory state with DHA omega-3, rebalancing the other omega fatty acids, and preventing future dietary brain inflammation.

Increasing the intake of omega-3's is an essential step, and must be performed to maximize the brain's natural capacity to restore proper neurological development by synaptic pruning and neuronal repair, and insure maximum recovery.

Our modern brains require a blend of omega-3 fatty acids which are the core nutrients that previous generations enjoyed in their food sources that are deficient in our food supply today.

There are three types of omega-3 that have different functions: DHA, EPA, and ALA. DHA is docosahexaenoic acid, EPA is eicosapentaenoic acid, and ALA is alpha-linolenic acid.

All three types of omega-3 are important but for this part of The Nemechek Protocol™ we focus on the DHA component in particular for its ability to aid in the repair of brain damage from inflammation and injury.

DHA is the only omega-3 fatty acid that penetrates the brain to any great extent and is found in variable amounts in fish oil.

Patients must supplement with the omega-3 DHA component in order to shift their primed microglia cells back into the microglia type that allows proper brain development and recovery from cumulative brain injury. There are no substitutes for the DHA component.

The amounts of daily omega-3 DHA that I use with my patients may be taken all at once, or they may be taken in divided doses throughout the day.

I always say that the best time of day for a parent to administer omega-3 to my patient is whatever time of day the parent will consistently remember to give it to their child.

The specific amount of accompanying EPA that is paired with the

DHA component in fish oil does not matter as much because the EPA component does not readily penetrate the central nervous system.

I personally prefer high concentration DHA fish oil pills or liquids that are available from NOW® Foods or Nordic Naturals®. These are the brands I have used with my patients that have resulted in success and autonomic dysfunction improvement or recovery.

But if these brands or a high concentration DHA fish oil pill is not readily available for my patient, I will then recommend they find any high-quality fish oil in liquid, capsule, or gummy form.

Cod liver oil also works well when supplementing omega-3 fatty acids, and it is dosed in the same manner as regular fish oil.

DHA and EPA Omega-3 Fatty Acid Supplementation from Fish Oil

The dosage of fish oil I recommend for my patients is based on their age and the severity of their inflammation.

I have found that different individuals have varying needs but in general terms, these are the starting doses I often use with patients.

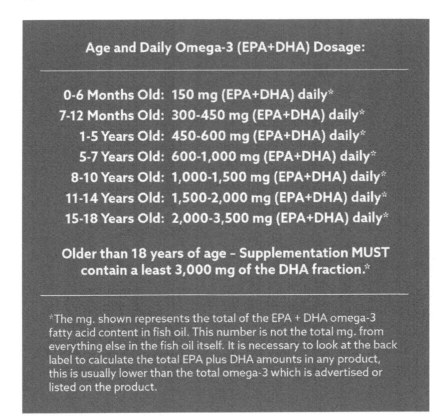

Age and Daily Omega-3 (EPA+DHA) Dosage:

0-6 Months Old: 150 mg (EPA+DHA) daily*
7-12 Months Old: 300-450 mg (EPA+DHA) daily*
1-5 Years Old: 450-600 mg (EPA+DHA) daily*
5-7 Years Old: 600-1,000 mg (EPA+DHA) daily*
8-10 Years Old: 1,000-1,500 mg (EPA+DHA) daily*
11-14 Years Old: 1,500-2,000 mg (EPA+DHA) daily*
15-18 Years Old: 2,000-3,500 mg (EPA+DHA) daily*

Older than 18 years of age – Supplementation MUST contain a least 3,000 mg of the DHA fraction.*

*The mg. shown represents the total of the EPA + DHA omega-3 fatty acid content in fish oil. This number is not the total mg. from everything else in the fish oil itself. It is necessary to look at the back label to calculate the total EPA plus DHA amounts in any product, this is usually lower than the total omega-3 which is advertised or listed on the product.

The fish oil amounts listed above are my basic starting dosages below. If, after several months of consistent EPA and DHA compliance there is no improvement in neurological function using the brands that I have suggested, I often will begin to double the dosage in my patients.

Pointers:

Does fish oil cause intestinal distress? Sometimes my patients may experience loose stools that can occur when first starting their fish oil. This is often due to their intestinal tract being irritated from bacterial overgrowth or not being able to absorb the sudden increase of oil being ingested.

If loose stools occur, I will have my patients stop their fish oil for two to three weeks until their intestinal function repairs itself.

After two or three weeks, my patients are allowed to restart their fish oil at a 1/4 of the full dose. They may slowly increase the dosage by adding another 1/4 of dose every one to two weeks until they reach the full dose. The reason for this is that by slowly increasing the amount of fish oil we essentially train the intestinal tract to increase its ability to absorb the fatty acid molecules.

Do I ever add vitamins or products in addition to fish oil in my patients? No. The addition of supplements such as glutamine, digestive enzymes, biofilm agents, or anti-fungal medications are not necessary for intestinal bacteria recovery from bacterial overgrowth or the absorption of fish oil.

Do I ever use fermented fish oil with my patients? No. I do not recommend fermented fish oils for my patients.

Do I ever use krill oil with my patients? No. Krill oil is a different molecule than the fish oil molecule. Our ancestors evolved on the shorter molecule that is found in fish oil, not on the longer molecule found in krill oil. I keep things in The Nemechek Protocol™ very simple and basic, I use the exact same molecules and core nutrients that used to keep our ancestor's brains strong and resilient.

Is there a vegetarian option if your patients are allergic to fish or do not want to ingest a fish byproduct? Maybe. There is algae-derived DHA which might be beneficial but as a doctor I have never witnessed any of my adult or child patients on any algae-derived DHA have any significant improvement. Autonomic improvement and recovery, medically thought to be impossible until I invented The Nemechek Protocol™ in my medical practice, has only been realized with marine-based DHA.

Can one form of omega-3 (EPA or ALA) substitute for the DHA from fish? No. Other forms of non-marine omega-3 fatty acids, such as flax oil (ALA), do not penetrate the central nervous system enough to have an impact on inflammation or microglia function.

Warning:

I never use any omega 3-6-9 combination products with my patients. The excessive amount of dietary omega-6 fatty acids are a large part of the problem with inflammation so I avoid them in my practice. Adding more omega-6 fatty acids of any sort may only serve to worsen the underlying inflammation.

Adults Age 18 or Older
ALA Omega-3 Supplementation
from Nuts, Flax, or Chia

The third component of omega-3 is ALA, (alpha-linolenic acid), which is plant-based omega-3. There is some research that suggests ALA may help small amounts of DHA penetrate into the brain, but at this time it is not known for certain.

My late teens and adult patients on The Nemechek Protocol™ take some form of daily supplementation of omega-3 ALA either from nuts (dry-roasted), flax, or ground chia seeds, as long as they are not allergic to any of those items.

If my patients chose to consume nuts as part of The Nemechek Protocol™, I instruct them to eat a minimum of ¼ cup of nuts per day. All tree nuts contain adequate supplies of ALA and these include almonds, pecans, pistachios, cashews, and walnuts.

Dry or roasted peanuts, which are legumes and are not tree nuts, are an acceptable ALA source as well. Dry or roasted peanuts are different than peanuts in other forms like peanut butters, which may contain some of the dietary omega-6 vegetables oils (soybean oil, cottonseed oil, grapeseed oil) that my patients are actively reducing.

If my patient decides to consume their ALA by flax seed or ground chia seeds, they will supplement with 1/2 to 1 tablespoon per day.

If they are consuming flax oil in liquid or in soft gel form, the amount is between 500 to 1,000 mg once daily.

STEP 3. REDUCTION OF DIETARY INTAKE OF OMEGA-6 FATTY ACIDS

Part of reducing pro-inflammatory cytokines on The Nemechek Protocol™ comes from a decrease in the patient's dietary intake of high concentration omega-6 fatty acid cooking oils.

This is done both by no longer cooking with them (vegetable oils, margarine, shortening), and by eliminating foods that contain high linoleic acid oils as ingredients.

I instruct my patients to avoid consuming food products that contain omega-6 fatty acids, and these are **prohibited**:

- Soy (Soybean) Oil
- Sunflower Oil
- Corn Oil
- Safflower Oil
- Cottonseed Oil
- Grapeseed Oil
- Peanut Oil
- Margarine
- Shortening

Foods containing soy milk or soy protein are allowed as long as they do not also list any of the prohibited oils on the label.

In these first stages of The Nemechek Protocol™ eliminating omega-6 oils from foods is often the most difficult thing for my patients to do. It is necessary for them to read the labels of all processed, store-bought foods.

If the food product contains any of those prohibited oils listed above, they must find a different brand or find one that contains an acceptable oil.

There are a few oils that have a healthier balance of omega-6 to omega-3 fatty acid ratio and these are **acceptable**:

- Canola Oil

- Coconut Oil
- Palm Kernel Oil

Once my patients start reading labels for omega-6 oils, it becomes clear to them the extent that these oils now appear in foods that they eat every day such as salad dressings and bread.

Omega-6 oils can be found in foods that we may otherwise consider to be clean, organic, and healthy. They even appear as ingredients in some dog foods.

Pointer:

I tell patients to memorize the three acceptable oils, it is easier than trying to memorize the prohibited oils.

I often say, "My patients *can*, have *can*ola oil".

Warning:

Some products will say that they contain either a prohibited or an acceptable oil (e.g. "may contain soybean oil or canola oil"). The consumer is left to wonder which oil is being used in the product. I personally err on the side of caution and avoid the products whose ingredients are not clear to me.

STEP 4. PREVENTION OF BRAIN AND SYSTEMIC INFLAMMATION FROM EXCESSIVE DIETARY LINOLEIC, ARACHIDONIC AND PALMITIC ACIDS

While on The Nemechek Protocol™, patients must make a consistent effort to avoid omega-6 in cooking oils and foods but also to protect themselves from omega-6 that they cannot control.

There are three specific acids I ask my patients to avoid in order to prevent brain inflammation are:

1. Linoleic acid is most commonly found in the unnatural vegetable oils added to the foods we purchased.

2. Arachidonic acid is found in elevated concentrations in dietary meats that are fed grains such as soy beans or corn.

3. Palmitic acid is found in high quantities in processed foods as well as grain fed foods.

These are types of things that patients find hard to control because they may not be able to see them on an ingredient label, they may not know what might have been fed to the meat or fish they eat, or they do not know what type of cooking oils are being used by a restaurant.

This is where a whole new type of protective omega fatty acid is introduced to my patients on The Nemechek Protocol™, and this is the omega-9 fatty acid that is found in authentic, domestic, extra virgin olive oil.

The use or consumption of omega-9 an essential step, and it must be performed on a regular basis in order to ensure maximum recovery.

Daily Supplementation with California Extra Virgin Olive Oil to Reduce Systemic Inflammation

In addition to decreasing the consumption of high concentration omega-6 fatty acid cooking oils as instructed, all of my patient's families are asked to cook their foods in domestic extra virgin olive oil (EVOO).

EVOO contains 70% oleic acid, and oleic acid not only blocks but it also reverses the underlying inflammation coming from excessive omega-6 fatty acid and palmitic acid toxicity.

Specifically, my patients are instructed to cook all of their home prepared foods in California sourced (see warning below on imported EVOO) extra virgin olive oil daily.

Several studies indicate that adults will benefit from consuming 2 tablespoons (30 ml) of extra virgin olive oil daily. But the daily doses for children are less clear.

For my patients who are children less that 5 years old, I believe that using EVOO when cooking foods should be an adequate amount. Starting at age 5, in addition to cooking with EVOO, my patients are given the following guidelines:

-Age 5 - 10 years, consume 1/2 a tablespoon a day.

-Age 11 - 18 years, consume 1 tablespoon per day.

-Age 19 years and older, consume 2 tablespoons per day.

Pointer:

EVOO may be mixed into a variety of liquids or taken by spoon. Some of my older patients cut the taste with a drop of balsamic or a drop of lemon juice.

Warning:

EVOO is a largely unregulated product and agricultural fraud or adulterated imported products is a great concern for my patients. Some olive oils may be diluted with a high percentage of soy oil or other vegetable oils, the very things we are trying to avoid.

Because of the high risk of purchasing fraudulent imported olive oils, patients on The Nemechek Protocol™ only use extra virgin olive oils certified by the California Olive Oil Council (go to www.cooc.com for more information).

There are a variety of tastes and flavors in the COOC certified oils, so I encourage families to experiment with different producers until they find one that their family prefers.

STEP 5. INDUCTION OF NEUROPLASTICITY

Neuroplasticity is the ability of the brain to form and reorganize synaptic connections. In other words, this is how the brain finds new pathways through neurons to perform certain tasks.

Because of the inflammatory stress they experience, all children with autism have impairment of neuroplasticity. This also contributes to their underlying developmental delay or arrest, as well as their cumulative brain injury.

Steps 1-4 all help restore natural neuroplasticity but additional steps can be taken to improve the brain's ability to create new neuronal connections required for normal functioning.

Many autistic children are already enrolled in these programs, and the neuro-cognitive improvement they experience is from the process of neuroplasticity. Some programs include:

- Vagus Nerve Stimulation (VNS)
- Applied Behavioral Analysis (ABA)
- Pivotal Response Therapy
- Verbal Behavior Therapy
- Sensory Integration Therapy

Vagus nerve stimulation (VNS) is a treatment that involves electrical stimulation of the Vagus nerve. The Vagus nerve is the 10th cranial nerve and carries information from the parasympathetic branch of the autonomic nervous system.

Neurological signals on the Vagus nerve travel both upwards into the brain and downwards to all the organs in the body. Signals traveling upwards are capable of inducing neuroplasticity while signals traveling downward improve organ function and help suppress abnormal levels of inflammation.

VNS results in suppression of inflammation as well as increased neuroplasticity especially when paired with a cognitive (speech, reading, mathematics training), sensory (integration therapy), or motor (physical therapy or gait training) activity.

Vagus Nerve Stimulation

My area of interest, and the focus of my internal medical practice, is in the dysfunction and recovery of the autonomic nervous system. I will describe the autonomic nervous system and my treatment invention in more detail, **The Nemechek Protocol™ for Autonomic Recov-**

ery, Patent Pending, (The Nemechek Protocol™ for Autism is only one part of my program) in Appendix I of this book.

For the purposes of this chapter, I am making you aware that the autonomic nervous system is an integral part of inflammation control for our brains and bodies.

Vagal nerve stimulation is a physician prescribed medical treatment that involves delivering very low electrical impulses to the Vagus Nerve. The Vagus nerve carries inflammation information in the parasympathetic branch of the autonomic nervous system.

Vagus nerve stimulators have been implanted in patients in the U.S. since the late 1990's, but it is also possible to stimulate the nerve externally. This is called bioelectric medicine. I use a portable Vagus nerve stimulator as part of The Nemechek Protocol™ that many of my adult patients and a few of my autistic patients use at home.

The use of transcutaneous (on the skin) Vagus nerve stimulation (tVNS) for 5-10 minutes per day is an extremely powerful and effective tool for suppression of inflammation as well as for the induction of neuroplasticity.

The suppression of inflammation within the brain improves the brain repair and neuronal pruning abilities of microglia.

I may add tVNS to a child's treatment a later stage in The Nemechek Protocol™ if there is no recovery. Once recovery has begun, tVNS treatment does not speed up or expand the breadth of a child's recovery and is not necessary. The use of tVNS is to trigger a change in patients who did not respond.

Individual patients of mine use different frequency settings and for different lengths of time, based on a number of factors that I take under consideration as their doctor.

It is possible for tVNS to cause harm if it is programmed or performed incorrectly.

I am a leading expert in the clinical application of tVNS and many of my patients travel to my office in Arizona to be prescribed a portable transcutaneous Vagus nerve stimulator they can use at home, with the ability to purchase replacement parts for the next year.

I do not prescribe or perform any other non-electrical methods of Vagus stimulation because I believe other methods to be ineffective at maintaining the healthy shift in microglia function.

Pointer:

Most of my autistic patients do not need tVNS. My most severe case of adult autism continues to improve year by year without using tVNS.

Warning:

tVNS is not readily available and requires management from a physician skilled in this methodology. No one should attempt this on their own because they could cause harm to their child.

Specific electrical settings and durations of time are required for safe and effective treatment.

7

RECOVERY AND PROBLEM SOLVING WITH THE NEMECHEK PROTOCOL

MINIMIZE VARIABLES

"Parents often ask, "How fast does it take for the brain to recover?"

The brain recovers as fast as hair grows. Everyday your hair looks the same length until, after a few months, you suddenly realize that you need a haircut."

— Dr. Patrick M. Nemechek, D.O.

THE PROCESS OF RECOVERY

The process of reversal and recovery of the key features of autism that I have seen in my patients begins with the awakening period. After the awakening period, a parent will see the full extent of the child's underlying developmental delay, brain injuries, and autonomic nervous system dysfunction. From this point going forward, normal neuronal pruning can begin the process of gradual neurological development and maturation.

All children with autism have some degree of developmental

delay underlying the stupor caused by propionic acid. The reversal of bacterial overgrowth with inulin or rifaximin results in the drop of the propionic acid and the reversal of the toxic encephalopathy. The drop usually results in a sudden improvement in function and awareness within a few weeks.

Despite these improvements in function and awareness with the drop in propionic acid, many children do not return to normal functioning because they still have some degree of underlying developmental delay (in some patients quite severe) as well as ADD, ADHD, sensory issues, or seizures. These children may also have chronic depression, anxiety, or aggressive behaviors due to unresolved past brain injuries.

As the drugged propionic state lifts, the parents will observe the child's present state of any underlying emotional, motor, and sensory development. Symptoms and behaviors might seem to be getting worse at this point, but this is not a worsening of autism.

The true extent of the child's developmental delay, brain injuries, and autonomic dysfunction might just be different than the parents had realized. Or the awakened child is finally able to express the symptoms of their injuries.

The child's remaining developmental delay or brain injuries are conditions that will take longer to reverse or recover, but month by month and then year by year, these things can slowly improve.

HOW EARLY CAN THE NEMECHEK PROTOCOL™ BE STARTED?

I recommend that people consult their pediatrician if their child is less than 12 months of age, or if there are any other concerning issues for a child of any age, prior to starting any new regimen.

In my patients, I believe the fish oil and inulin components of The Nemechek Protocol™ should be started at the earliest sign of any developmental problems in a child.

The fish oil supplementation may be started in newborns or early in a child's life, especially if the child's mother has some signs of bacterial overgrowth herself.

The inulin supplementation may be started with any sign of chronic colic, constipation, diarrhea, or reflux.

AGE OF THE PATIENT AND LENGTH OF TIME

The age of the patient and the length of time they have been under the influence of propionic acid are two variables in the recovery process.

It is important to understand that the brain recovery process takes time, consistent effort, and may greatly depend on the age of the child. Younger patients might initially respond faster, but I have seen significant progress in young adults with autism as well.

I believe the reasons for different recoveries and rates of improvement in my patients are because the brain of an older child will have experienced prolonged bacterial overgrowth and inflammation, while a younger child's brain has not.

Older children may also have multiple unresolved brain injuries due to the primed microglia cycle of more damage with less repair throughout their years.

I provide care for two teenage non-verbal autistic boys (14 and 16 years of age), and although they showed signs of continual improvement they took about four or five months to begin speaking.

In terms of speech and communication, younger patients may start speaking within a few weeks while teenagers might take four to six months.

One 23-year-old patient did not start speaking until she was eight or nine months into her treatment with me.

But strikingly, and even in the most severe cases I have worked with, the young adults have had a noticeable improvement in their awareness of their surroundings within the first few weeks.

THE AWAKENING PERIOD

The first change I see in recovery during the first few weeks with my patients is due to the initial decline of the toxic effects of the propionic acid on their brains. This is what I call "the awakening period".

It helps to view a child with autism as a child who has been on a sedative such as Valium. All of their behaviors will be subdued, they may sleep more, they may seem calm, they may not be coherent, they may not talk, and they may not be aware of their surroundings.

In the case of autism, the sedative is the propionic acid made by bacteria in the child's own intestinal tract.

Reversing the bacterial overgrowth essentially removes the sedative from their body, and the child becomes more cognitively alert.

Children in the awakening period are more aware of their surroundings. They are often more tolerant of being touched or held, and are often more willing to approach someone and be physically closer to them. They may also be more active and energetic, communicate more, and often sleep less.

After the first few weeks of the awakening period, recovery rates are highly variable due to the degree of developmental delay underlying each patient's toxic encephalopathy state.

If the inflammatory cytokine process has been going on since birth, the child will be obviously experiencing difficulties unlike a child who is developing normally until their regressive event at eighteen months for instance.

If the inflammation is mild, the developmental delay often is relatively mild, and the children often regain function rather quickly.

With very early and intense inflammation, there can be so much developmental delay or arrest that the child may labeled mentally retarded. In spite of this, I have children under my care who fit this description and they are recovering as anticipated. It may take longer for them but I do not see any hurdles that are impassable.

THE TRUE EXTENT OF BRAIN DYSFUNCTION

But if the child also has underlying brain injuries from physical, emotional or inflammatory traumas, the parents may see more angry outbursts, hyperactivity, anxiety, and stimulation behavior after the awakening period.

And because the child will very often also have underlying developmental delay, parents will observe immature behaviors that do not match the current age of the child.

Parents may observe a child who is the size of a 14-year old who emotionally behaves as a 3-year old, or a child who can type but not speak, or a teenager that has the coordination of a 7-year old.

Developmental delay may occur in one region of the brain much more than in another so the potential combinations of developmental mismatches in children is vast.

The overriding point is that the change of behaviors after the awakening period is not worsening of underlying problems it is finally a glimpse of the true degree of underlying damage and developmental delay, because the sedative that dampened their overall behavior is finally gone. The children are not worse, they are finally awake.

For some parents, this stage may be more challenging than others because the underlying behaviors are more disruptive to the household.

After reducing bacterial overgrowth, new development and repair is dependent on consistently reducing inflammation with fish oil, California EVOO, and removing the omega-6 vegetable oils from the diet.

These behaviors should improve because a child's brain is remarkably capable of recovering.

My 23-year old non-verbal ASD young adult patient was finally able to start speaking in both Spanish and English after eight months but only after going through a period of angry outbursts on the school bus, experiencing increased anxiety when she was sitting still, and after going through spells of having tantrums in the grocery store.

Once her propionic levels declined she developmentally had tantrums like any other 3-year-old in the grocery store when her parents would tell her to put an item back on the shelf.

Her angry outbursts and anxiety were from lingering autonomic nervous system dysfunction that triggered her "fight or flight" feelings if she sat still for too long.

But now her brain has developed and her autonomic nervous system has recovered from whatever developmental deficiencies or brain injuries that had caused these behaviors.

THE PACE OF RECOVERY

The important point to remember is that a child's brain has an enormous capacity to continue the path of development once the inflammation is consistently controlled.

Neuronal and synaptic pruning will re-initiate, and according to the developmental delay literature, children can catch-up about two to three months of development for every one calendar month.

In my experience recovery does seem to advance this fast, if not faster.

I am frequently asked what else might someone do to speed the healing.

I tell parents to think of the brain repair process like someone wanting to speed up the recovery of their broken arm. A broken arm will not heal any faster by doing anything "extra".

I also tell parents not to compare their child's behavior today with yesterday, instead compare them to how they were several months ago, or when they first started as my patient.

Improvements may be slow or plateau at times, so I also encourage them to hang in there and to continue with the fish oil. But if the child has no significant improvement within the first two months I will begin to make adjustments to their fish oil.

I generally have the parents begin to double the dosage of my patient's omega-3 fatty acids.

And if my patient still does not improve, particularly if they were born with autism, I may add bioelectric Vagus Nerve Stimulation to their treatment in an effort to further decrease cytokine production and inflammation. The majority of my patients, however, do not need this treatment step.

HISTAMINE RELEASE

Some of my patient's parents ask about histamine release, and it is always necessary to discuss histamine reactions with your child's physician(s).

Histamine is a chemical released from a white blood cell called a mast cell, and is released when the white blood cell is activated. Activation of white blood cells is commonly referred to as inflammation.

A healthy histamine response by mast cells requires a balance between the production and removal of histamine.

Excessive histamine reactions are due to the excessive production of histamine, excessive dietary intake of histamine, or the inadequate removal of histamine from the tissues due to a genetic deficiency of diamine oxidase (DAO).

Sources of Excessive Histamine:

1. True Allergic Reaction to a Substance
2. Increased Dietary Intake of Histamine
3. Inflammatory Release of Histamine from Mast Cells
4. Decreased Clearance of Histamine due to DAO Deficiency

A clinical reaction from excessive histamine due to any or all of the aforementioned mechanisms may cause headaches, rapid heart rate, hives, itching, diarrhea and low blood pressure.

In children with autism, increases in stimming, aggression, or headaches are frequently reported by their parents. Each of these mechanisms can lead to a clinical reaction for increased histamine levels within the blood stream.

True allergic reactions to foods or medications are not uncommon, and they can cause a release of histamine. Sometimes a true allergic scenario can be life-threatening, as is the case with peanut or walnut allergies.

Increased histamine levels can also occur if an individual has a genetic mutation leading to a deficiency in the diamine oxidase (DAO), the enzyme responsible for degrading and removing histamine from the intestinal tissues. These mutations are somewhat rare within the general population.

Many people believe that fish itself is high in histamine and this is incorrect. Their belief may be based on observing someone who was taking fish oil or eating fish might have a histamine reaction.

The histamine reaction that most people experience is not from histamine within the fish but is actually produced by bacteria in inadequately preserved and improperly refrigerated fish.

This problem used to be called scromboid fish poisoning. The term "histamine fish poisoning" is now considered more appropriate because many cases are from nonscombroid fish. Examples include mahi-mahi (dolphin fish), amberjack, herring, sardine, anchovy, and bluefish.

The reaction from fish resembles an allergic reaction but it is actually caused by bacterially-generated toxins in the fish's tissues.

If fish oil is manufactured from tainted fish, one might expect the fish oil to contain higher levels of histamine and other toxins.

I believe the primary causes of histamine reactions noted in autism originate from either poor quality fish oil and/or from an excessive inflammatory stimulation of the mast cells surrounding the small intestine with a release of histamine.

The two factors of such a reaction are (1) from the increased inflammation from bacterial translocation (leaky gut) due to bacterial overgrowth, and (2) from the loss of the autonomic nervous system inflammatory reflex due to cumulative brain injury.

The autonomic inflammatory reflex, also known as the vagus inflammatory reflex, refers to control of the immune cells (including mast cells) surrounding the small intestine by both the parasympathetic and sympathetic branches of the autonomic nervous system.

Chronic damage to this inflammation control mechanism commonly occurs with cumulative brain injury.

The Nemechek Protocol™ minimizes excessive histamine reactions through a few basic tenets:

1. My patients always use a high-quality fish oil. Nordic Naturals and NOW Foods have excellent reputations and they consistently prove to be of high quality when tested by independent laboratories.

2. If there is a history of histamine reactions in my patient, I delay starting supplementation with fish oil for 2-3 weeks after the initiation of inulin or after treatment with rifaximin to allow the intestinal tract to heal. Allowing the intestinal tract to heal may prevent leakage of histamine possibly contained within food, and would lessen the release of histamine from the inflammation associated with bacterial translocation (leaky gut).

3. If symptoms are persistent in spite of this, I consider the use of single or dual histamine blockade therapy with an

H1-allergy anti-histamine and/or and H2-antacid antihistamine.

4. I would then consider rebalancing the intestinal tract with rifaximin in a younger patient if there is suspicion that bacterial overgrowth is not adequately suppressed with inulin alone over time.

OVER FOCUSING AND MISINTERPRETING

Some changes during or after the awakening period may be in the child's skin condition or in the movement or speed of the digestive tract.

One of the misconceptions I encounter with patients is that other than an occasional mild skin rash after rebalancing the gut, the "yeast effects" reported by many parents are not from yeast. Changes in the skin, stool, and behavior are from the shifting of the bacteria and the extent of the underlying issues.

In patients with autism, I like seeing signs that they have a reduction in anxiety (better sleep, less anxiety, less stimming), are more in touch with their surroundings (improved eye-to-eye contact, recognizing the arrival of a familiar person) or are more awake or alert (less napping, wake up earlier, increased mental activity and engagement). These are signs to me that the propionic acid levels are dropping.

Some parents will over-focus on a smaller issue (constipation, giggling more, waking up earlier, holding hands over ears, moodiness, etc.) and interpret such thing as being bad or negative.

These things can seem quite strange but will resolve with a little developmental recovery over time. Over-focusing in this manner may cause a parent to miss the bigger picture that this is just one step in the child's gradual improvement.

This is the transition of a child with developmental delay affected by propionic acid changing into a child not affected by propionic acid.

BEHAVIOR-AGE MISMATCH

Parents need to anticipate that their children's emotional maturity generally will not match their physical age during recovery.

They may have an autistic child who is 6, 12, or 24 years old but behaves as if they are a 2-year-old child. They must do their best to be patient during this difficult time because in a few more months a child who behaved liked a 2-year-old child may begin behaving as if they are 3 or 4 years old.

In a few months after that they may progress to the behavior of a 5 or 6-year-old. So on and so forth.

My 23-year-old patient that learned to talk after eight months on this protocol initially behaved as if she were a 3-year-old. Her parents reported that she had been around the age of four when her condition had become worse as a little girl.

But within six months these tantrums had stopped and she began talking and behaving more like a 5-year-old girl (playing dress up, sharing toys, etc.).

Children with autism have the ability to developmentally recover at a rate that is about two to three months for every calendar month that inflammation is lowered, but emotional maturity in different individuals may happen in fits and starts.

CONSTIPATION, STIMMING AND AUTONOMIC DYSFUNCTION

The autonomic nervous system (ANS) is a large portion of the nervous system that controls and coordinates all organ function, hormonal production, and most of the immune system.

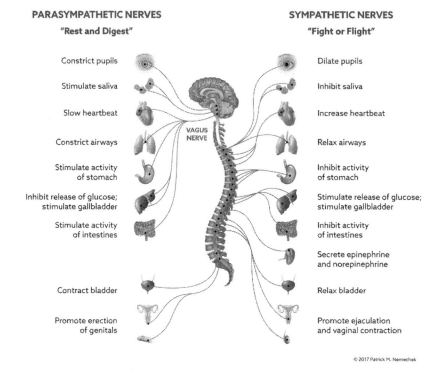

PARASYMPATHETIC NERVES
"Rest and Digest"

Constrict pupils
Stimulate saliva
Slow heartbeat
Constrict airways
Stimulate activity of stomach
Inhibit release of glucose; stimulate gallbladder
Stimulate activity of intestines

Contract bladder
Promote erection of genitals

VAGUS NERVE

SYMPATHETIC NERVES
"Fight or Flight"

Dilate pupils
Inhibit saliva
Increase heartbeat
Relax airways
Inhibit activity of stomach
Stimulate release of glucose; stimulate gallbladder
Inhibit activity of intestines
Secrete epinephrine and norepinephrine
Relax bladder
Promote ejaculation and vaginal contraction

© 2017 Patrick M. Nemechek

The same inflammatory process that prevents the brain from properly developing will also prevent the brain from repairing damage to the autonomic nervous system that occurs with head banging, accidental falls, intense emotional traumas, or inflammatory trauma from surgery, allergy testing, or adverse vaccine reaction.

The residual damage from prior injuries will add to the damage from new injuries in a process known as cumulative brain injury (CBI).

The cumulative brain injuries will ultimately lead to enough autonomic nervous system damage that the child will experience symptoms.

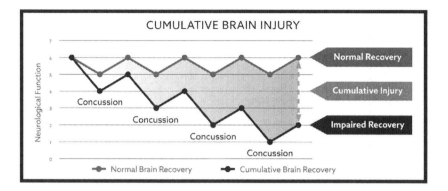

A very common problem after the reversal of bacterial overgrowth is the appearance of constipation in children. The brain controls the movement of the digestive tract, like a conveyor belt, through the autonomic nervous system.

From an autonomic viewpoint, constipation is the inability of the nervous system to push the contents of the stool forward on that conveyor belt.

Understanding the mechanics that move the digestive tract helps parents understand the changes that they see in my patient during treatment of the bacterial overgrowth. Bacterial overgrowth may lead to either constipation or diarrhea (an increased rate of stool production), or both.

If a child has an increased rate of stool production from bacterial overgrowth (i.e., diarrhea) while at the same time has inadequate forward stool propulsion from autonomic nervous system damage (i.e. constipation), they may seem to have a normal stool pattern.

The parents do not understand that this normal pattern may just be from two opposite imbalances.

This is why once the bacterial overgrowth is rebalanced and corrected with either inulin or rifaximin, the child's constipation suddenly seems to 'be caused by' these therapies.

But in fact, what actually happens is that the diarrhea simply resolved thereby making the underlying neurological problem (constipation) more obvious.

The underlying neurological problem (constipation) is something that slowly improves as the patient diligently takes their fish oil, EVOO, and reduces their dietary omega-6 oils.

These simple and effective tools in The Nemechek Protocol ™ steadily shift the patient's microglia into repair mode, reduce brain inflammation, and stimulates brain stem cell production.

When these things occur, the repair of the autonomic nervous system also begins in earnest. It is the improvement of autonomic nervous system function that allows the digestive conveyor belt to move more naturally again.

Fortunately, the nervous system is capable of recovering as long as the brain inflammation is adequately controlled with fish oil, EVOO, reduced omega-6, and Vagus nerve stimulation when appropriate.

ANXIETY, STIMMING, AND AUTONOMIC DYSFUNCTION

Another common problem from autonomic nervous system dysfunction is the inability of the child to properly regulate blood pressure and oxygen delivery into the brain. This is referred to as cerebral hypoperfusion.

The low oxygen levels in the brain from cerebral hypoperfusion are common causes of headaches, lightheadedness, dizziness, increased levels of hunger or thirst, poor concentration, chronic fatigue, and anxiety in the children.

Sometimes the low oxygen levels in the brain may cause a rapid rise in a stress hormone called noradrenaline. Noradrenaline is the body's primary "fight or flight" hormone that comes from the sympathetic branch of the autonomic nervous system.

The release of this hormone may cause children to become aggressive, angry, physically violent or anxious, panicky, and overwhelmed.

This noradrenaline rush may also result in some children having a temporary increase in self-stimulatory (stimming) and repetitive behavior, tantrums, and clinginess.

I see these problems in my autonomic dysfunction patients frequently. Increasing my patient's hydration or boosting their dietary intake of salt can help with some of their milder low brain oxygen symptoms.

Low brain oxygen symptoms and emotional outbursts may occur when the children are sitting still for prolonged periods of time.

Common examples of this are acting in an aggressive manner (hitting, yelling, or biting) on the school bus, while riding in a car, or while sitting in class.

Simple ways to help boost blood pressure and oxygen delivery to the brain includes allowing them to move around a little so their muscles constrict and push blood upwards against gravity. This may be done by getting them to stand up, walk around, or ride a bicycle.

For more serious cases that are not manageable by salt, hydration, and physical activity I recommend an evaluation by a neurologist or physician who has experience treating patients with autonomic nervous system dysfunction. There are medications that can boost blood pressure and help shut off these symptoms.

Over time as the brain recovers, these types of medications can be tapered off as the autonomic nervous system damage repairs itself.

SUPPLEMENTS AND PRESCRIPTION MEDICATIONS

I believe that a child who is under the direct supervision of a physician who prescribes medications and supplements should always consult with that prescribing physician about all of the medicines and other products that the child is given.

No prescribed medicines or supplements should ever be reduced or stopped without the permission and upon the direction of that physician.

I also believe that children are being over-treated with an enormous number of supplements for oxidative stress, mitochondrial defects, digestion, biofilm, yeast overgrowth, and other genetically-induced metabolic disturbances.

Although many of those types of supplements may have improved something, they do not have a significant impact on the overall pattern of bacterial overgrowth, brain injury symptoms, and autonomic nervous system dysfunction that are such key features of autism and developmental delay.

The Nemechek Protocol ™ does not use any of those types of products because I see positive results without using them.

In my experience, they do not solve those target problems. If they *could* have fixed these problems, they *would* have fixed these problems.

The reasons why are because those types of products are often only addressing the downstream effects of the much larger and overwhelming issue of metabolic inflammation.

Metabolic inflammation is the term used to describe the broad adverse effects that the chronic elevation of pro-inflammatory cytokines has on cellular function. Metabolic inflammation must be persistently lowered to have lasting cellular improvement.

I often speak of metabolic inflammation like it is water that is flooding a valley because the dam upstream is broken and it no longer holds back the water. When the dam breaks the homes and fields downstream of the dam become flooded from the excessive flow of water.

The water in my example is meant to represent the massive release of pro-inflammatory cytokines associated with bacterial overgrowth and the dietary omega-3 and omega-6 fatty acid imbalance.

Certain efforts, such as placing sandbags around a home or pumping water out of a basement, may provide some benefit to the flooded area but they do not address the primary problem which is the broken dam.

Sand bags and basement pumps are similar to many of the supplements used to address mitochondrial dysfunction or the depletion of antioxidants.

The real problem remains. The dam needs to be repaired and once that occurs, the sand bags and basement pumps are no longer required.

Once there is a reduction of metabolic inflammation with The Nemechek Protocol ™ in my patients, I see the need for supplements addressing mitochondrial dysfunction and antioxidant depletion disappear.

Warning:

In regard to all prescription medications or prescription supplements (e.g. leucovorin), parents should never under any circumstance reduce or stop those without first consulting the prescribing physician.

HIGH OMEGA-3, LOW OMEGA-6 OVERALL RATIO IS WHAT COUNTS

The most important aspect in reducing omega-6 fatty acid toxicity seems to be in the relative balance of our dietary ratio of omega-6 to omega-3.

It is the sum of the omega-6 to omega-3 ratio in all of our foods that really matters, and not whether any one particular food source contains any omega-6.

An equal 1 to 1 ratio of omega-6 to omega-3 is what our ancestors consumed. Throughout history that equal ratio kept their brains and nervous systems healthy and capable of repair.

The human body functions better with an omega-6 to omega-3 ratio around 1 - 2.5 of omega- 6 to 1 omega-3 (1-2.5:1). Today our estimated omega-6 intake is twenty times over our omega-3 intake (20:1).

Consumption of fish oil, EVOO, and the elimination of omega-6 oils from the diet is adequate to normalize the unhealthy ratio.

UNDERSTANDING BACTERIAL TERMINIOLOGY

Our understanding about the diversity of microbes living within human intestinal tract is rapidly expanding, and a few phrases (dysbiosis, SIBO, and bacterial overgrowth) may seem similar but are all slightly different from each other.

Dysbiosis is a general term referring to any change in the blend of living microbes within the intestinal tract. It does not specifically apply to only bacteria and it may refer to viruses, protozoan, or archaebacteria.

In addition to an imbalance of one type or species of microorganism to another, dysbiosis may also refer to the absence of certain species thought to normally inhabit the human intestinal tract. The extinction or loss of species is referred to as low biodiversity.

SIBO (small intestinal bacterial overgrowth) implies the patient has an overgrowth of bacteria that abnormally produces hydrogen or methane in a breath test when fed sugar.

SIBO may also refer to an abnormally high concentration of bacteria within a certain amount of fluid taken from the small intestine. Getting a sample of intestinal fluid is a complicated medical procedure that is done at research facilities.

This procedure, which requires a long endoscope, tells the concentration of bacteria within the small intestine. This is considered the "gold standard" test for determining bacterial overgrowth.

It is important to note that a patient can have bacterial overgrowth as noted on this concentration test but still have a negative breath test.

In this context, the phrase "bacterial overgrowth" implies an overgrowth of bacteria within the small intestine regardless of the status of the breath test.

Within my practice, I stopped using SIBO breath testing on my patients to determine overgrowth because unacceptably high false positive and false negative results make it clinically useless.

I also stopped using SIBO breath tests because of the lack of correlation between it and the small intestinal concentration test.

I also do not recommend that my patients undergo the concentration test as it is expensive, it is relatively unavailable, and it is unnecessary in order to achieve improvement using The Nemechek Protocol™.

By definition all children with autism have bacterial overgrowth, so why perform a test when we already know the answer.

My experience has shown me that I must attempt to reverse any level of overgrowth, whether the breath test was positive or negative, if I want to restore the brain's ability to repair itself and restore neuronal pruning.

In order to reverse the damaging effect of autism, bacterial balance must be restored or the children simply fail to improve.

THE MISCONCEPTION OF FEEDING "BAD BACTERIA" AND YEAST, FEAR OF INULIN

It is difficult to imagine the hundreds of thousands of bacteria down in our digestive tract that are causing our brains and bodies so much trouble. Common questions from parents of my patients are whether inulin feeds "bad bacteria" and yeast.

Inulin is a safe prebiotic fiber that produces enough bacterial rebalancing, propionic acid reduction, and inflammation reduction to allow a child to become more alert and restart the process of neuronal pruning and development.

I generally recommend starting with inulin in patients who are children because it is effective, inexpensive, and does not require a prescription to obtain. Inulin is widely available from a number of manufacturers.

Inulin is also appealing as a natural fiber that many parents prefer who are understandably fearful of using any more antibiotics.

If my patient's parents are worried about using inulin because of the fear of "bad bacteria", I recommend they use rifaximin and eliminate the bacterial overgrowth altogether.

This moves them beyond the issue of "good" and "bad" bacteria that seem to be holding people back from starting my regimen. Rifaximin seems to work as well as inulin in children.

The conclusion that increased stimming, less sleeping, or increased anxiety is from inulin feeding "bad" bacteria such as Klebsiella are obvious concerns of these parents.

I am not saying this is impossible but I do not believe that to be the case with inulin. I have not seen any indication that inulin increases bacterial overgrowth in any of my patients. I believe there are several reasons for this.

The first reason is that inulin's main effect is within the lumen of the small intestine where bacteria digest inulin through a process referred to as fermentation.

The primary effect is the production of the healthy short chain fatty acid known as butyric acid. Only small amounts of inulin pass through to the colon.

The second reason why I do not believe inulin feeds bad bacteria or yeast is that a significant increase in pathogenic bacteria, or overgrowth of bacteria, would almost certainly cause an increase in diarrhea, stool frequency, abdominal cramping, reflux, and eczema.

I do not see those reactions in my patients, in fact I see a general reversal of those symptoms with the use of inulin.

If the intestinal (not neurological or behavioral) symptoms were to worsen on inulin, I would probably suggest that the inulin be discontinued and prescribe rifaximin for my patient.

Remember, the development of constipation with the use of inulin is a sign of underlying autonomic nervous system dysfunction from developmental and cumulative brain injury that typically reverses after a few months of diligent fish oil, EVOO, and a reduction in dietary omega-6 oils.

The third reason why I do not believe that inulin feeds bad bacteria or yeast is that propionic acid has a sedating effect on children, almost as if the children had been taking Valium or Xanax. Therefore, once inulin reverses the bacterial overgrowth and the propionic acid levels decline, I see the children come out of their stupor.

Their different behavior during or after the awakening period is the result of their pre-existing and underlying developmental abnormalities, cumulative brain injuries, and autonomic dysfunction.

I do not believe their behavior is from any toxic effect of inulin, as I have seen these behaviors improve or stop over time while the patient is on their continued inulin.

A fourth reason why I do not believe that inulin feeds bad bacteria or yeast is that the detection of pathogenic bacteria such as Klebsiella in the stool (a sample of bacteria within the colon not the small intestine) by no means suggests that these bacteria are present within the small intestine where inulin has its main effect.

The detection of pathogenic bacteria such as *Klebsiella pneuomiae* or *Clostridium difficle* are commonly found in asymptomatic patients and are essentially harmless. Their growth is kept in check by a healthy balance of other bacteria which is further bolstered with inulin.

In addition, some parents are worried about overgrowth of candida. I agree that candida and other yeasts (also known as fungi) inhabit the intestinal tract but recent in-depth studies demonstrate that yeast (fungal) overgrowth does not occur in autism.

The symptoms that have been misattributed to candida or yeast are instead the consequence of bacterial overgrowth.

Finally, while the observations of clinical improvement after the reduction of sugars (think GF/CF, FODMAPS, GAPS) are true, these are also misattributed to yeast instead of the bacterial overgrowth for which we now have mounting evidence.

INTESTINAL SYMPTOMS AND STOOL TESTING

When children are experiencing occasional intestinal issues, I always consider whether something else that is more common might have caused their intestinal symptoms. The things that I consider include a viral infection, an injury, an adverse vaccine reaction, or tainted food.

Reactions to those kinds of things should resolve within one to two weeks without necessitating a discontinuation of inulin in my patients.

I always eliminate probiotics, digestive aids, multivitamins, herbal remedies, and fermented foods other than yogurt in my patients on The Nemechek Protocol ™.

Occasionally my patients may develop some diarrhea, loose stools, or an oily film in the stool. These things generally occur for two reasons.

The first reason is that their intestinal tract is injured or stressed from the bacterial overgrowth. Their intestinal tract will begin to repair itself within two to three weeks after starting the inulin.

My patients do not need any special "gut-healing" supplements or special diets for those issues.

The second reason is that their intestines are not accustomed to absorbing the types of oils used on The Nemechek Protocol™. The intestinal tract alters its ability to absorb oils depending on the amount of oils in the person's diet.

To improve oil absorption in my patients, I first decrease their amounts of fish oil and EVOO to a lower dose that does not cause them any problems.

Then, I will slowly increase their dose a little every week until reaching the full dose in about three to four weeks.

I often have to explain and clarify to my patients that there is no such thing as "yeast effects" or "yeasty behaviors". The growing body of scientific research shows that there is no overgrowth from yeast in children with autism.

When comparing autistic and non-autistic children, microbiome studies consistently show suppressed levels of *Bifidobacterium* and elevated *Lactobacillus* bacteria while showing similar levels of yeast and other bacteria.

For many years, the symptoms and problems in adults and kids that were thought to be coming from yeast (fungus, candida) were actually coming from their bacterial overgrowth for the most part.

Testing the stool for bacteria and yeast is commonly performed by other practitioners and I urge a word of caution to my patients at their interpretation.

A stool sample comes from the colon which contains a very different blend of bacteria and yeast when compared to the small intestine where bacterial overgrowth actually occurs. Bacteria data from the distal colon is not particularly useful in determining what is going on in the small intestine.

On rare occasion, parasites (protozoans or helminths) are detected in the stool specimen. These might need to be treated depending on the organism found, the nature of the patient's symptoms, and the potential adverse effects of the treatment.

THE RISK OF RUNNING UNNECESSARY TESTS

By the time they come to my office, many of my patients have been misled, over-charged, and even harmed physically and emotionally by excessive and unnecessary laboratory (enzymes, food intolerance, metabolites, genetic panels) or physical (CT/MRI scans, EEG, etc.) testing.

Instead of spending time with patients to conduct a proper historical intake and physical exam, the modern era of medicine has seen an excessive dependence on the ordering of a wide variety of tests to help determine the cause of the patient's symptoms.

The traditional and most effective method of diagnostics in medicine is a thorough history and examination to determine the most probable cause of a person's symptoms.

As an internal medicine doctor, I was taught, and I believe, that a clinician should not order any testing until they have determined the one or two conditions that are most likely responsible for the patient's symptoms. Any tests that are run should be specific to either rule in or rule out these conditions.

Broad panels of tests should be avoided to limit expense and confusion in the patient's care. And certain tests such as colonoscopies, MRI scans, or EEG may also cause a child emotional distress.

Testing that requires general anesthesia may also present an opportunity for the worsening or the relapse of bacterial overgrowth.

Broad panels of tests for random things that do not change the patient's course of care should also be avoided. The question that I ask is whether the test outcome will change the course of treatment that I prescribe.

Part of my job is to be certain the tests will change the outcome of care before exposing my patients to more potential trauma.

RESTRICTING FOODS IN THE DIET

I do not restrict any foods in the diet when I treat my patients with The Nemechek Protocol™ other that those foods causing allergic reactions (peanuts, walnuts, etc.) and obvious intolerance (when milk causes diarrhea, etc.)

The benefits that occur in autistic patients after starting any diet that restricts carbohydrates (GAPS, FODMAPS, gluten, casein, etc.) is from a relative, non-specific decrease in the overall bacterial load within the intestinal tract.

The bulk of intestinal bacteria thrive on carbohydrates, and a decrease in bacterial counts occurs with a decrease in dietary carbohydrates.

If a child has been on a restrictive diet of some sort prior to starting The Nemechek Protocol™, it is fine to start reintroducing the restricted foods a few weeks after starting the inulin or after completing the course of rifaximin.

Obvious exceptions to this are foods such as peanuts that may have caused a severe allergic reaction previously in the child. These should never be re-introduced. If there are any questions about the severity of past food reactions, I recommend the parent discuss this with their physician.

Unfortunately, many children have developed their own limited pattern of food preferences. This can be very frustrating and is very worrisome for parents.

With time, this issue slowly resolves on its own but it might take months before the food preferences expand.

Gluten intolerance occurs because of an abnormal inflammatory reaction against gluten. This inflammatory reaction is a result of parasympathetic weakness of the autonomic nervous system and is not related to bacterial translocation (leaky gut).

Fortunately, I have seen as the child's brain starts recovering, the autonomic nervous system recovers, and gluten intolerance often slowly resolves without needing to remain on a gluten-free diet.

PHYSICAL, OCCUPATIONAL AND SPEECH THERAPIES

I do not think there is any problem continuing any form of occupational or physical therapy while a patient is on The Nemechek Protocol™.

In fact, PT/OT of any kind will help stimulate neuroplasticity, which is the process through which the brain develops new neuronal pathways to perform certain tasks and accelerates overall recovery.

MONITORING PROPIONIC ACID LEVELS

Although there are tests available that can measure propionic acid levels in the blood stream and urine, there are no set standards which we can use to determine if a level is too high or low.

Furthermore, there are a variety of metabolic variants of propionic acid (3HHA, 3HPA, HPHPA) and no one really knows whether or not they can be used as a marker for autism.

If a child under my care has any features resembling autism, any spectral disorder, ADD/ADHD, a mood disorder, or any form of developmental delay I will start them on The Nemechek Protocol™ because with any of these diagnoses the patient has a good chance of improvement or recovery regardless of a propionic-related test result.

If you go back and look at my flow chart "Autism and Other Childhood Developmental Disorders: The Steps to Recovery" the fourth chart in Chapter 3, you will see that the primed microglia and the inflammation will impair synaptic pruning and prevent the repair of neuronal injuries in children with both non-autistic issues (developmental delay, ADD, ADHD, mood disorders) and in mild to severe autistic children.

We already know that the non-autistic child will not have the propionic acid effects, while the autistic child will. My treatment of both children is the same, with or without the presence of propionic acid.

Take for example a child with severe developmental delay from a form of bacterial overgrowth that does not produce propionic acid.

Their test results for propionic acid would be normal (or negative) but their developmental delay would still recover after rebalancing their intestinal bacteria and omega fatty acids issues.

THE GENETIC WILDCARD IN RECOVERY

The underlying wild card for recovery while on The Nemechek Protocol™ is what genes might have been activated by the elevated levels of pro-inflammatory cytokines, and what the activated gene might do to the neurological impairment of that child's brain.

The inflammatory environment that prevents normal synaptic pruning and recovery from brain injury may also triggers the litany of genes being found in autism.

Inflammatory cytokines abnormally produced by the mother are affecting the child's nervous system within the womb. And then the imbalance of intestinal bacteria of the child, as well as high omega-6 food sources, continue to fuel the inflammatory process within the child after birth.

These inflammatory cytokines are the primary process through which the genes within the DNA that had been dormant for thousands of years in the child's ancestors are finally activated, begin altering how cells function, and contribute to the overall variety of neurological and behavioral characteristics that manifest in autism.

Many children with autism will often undergo genetic testing to help focus the diagnosis of their developmental disorder. But demonstrating there is a gene for a particular condition doesn't mean it is necessarily active.

A common example is that many people with brown eyes may be carrying a gene for blue eyes. They have the gene but it has not been activated. Current estimates suggest that only 20% of patients may exhibit features related to abnormal genes.

If any individual carries a gene for a particular condition, it is not a guarantee that the gene is or will become active because much of the activation is dependent on the inflammation cascade.

There is also additional evidence that a significant reduction in the inflammatory cascade may result in an active gene being switched off.

THE OTHER CHILDREN IN THE FAMILY

The imbalance of a child's intestinal bacteria bacterial has its genesis in the maternal lineage of your family. Most of my patients provide a family history suggesting intestinal dysbiosis began a few generations prior to the child with autism.

Each sequential mother's inherited bacterial blend is further disrupted by antibiotics, preservatives, pesticides, and then passed on to their children. The process then continues as the young children are again exposed to the same disrupting agents.

Unless a mother of an autistic child was specifically treated for bacterial overgrowth (rifaximin, inulin, FMT), it is highly likely the children born after the autistic child will also have bacterial overgrowth, and be susceptible to the chronically inflammatory and damaging primed-microglia.

"What to do?" is the million-dollar question at this point.

The threat of injury from the vaccine is real as is the danger of not being vaccinated against measles, a potentially deadly infectious disease which we have no treatment for.

It is important that to realize that it is the unstable intestinal bacteria that triggers the cascade resulting in autism, many developmental disorders as well as cumulative brain injury.

Vaccination is only one of several events that can push an 'unhealthy but not yet autistic bacterial blend' into a 'full propionic acid producing, inflammation autism-inducing blend.'

In addition to vaccines, antibiotics, surgeries, anesthetic, concussions, intestinal infections from parasites or viruses all can push the bacterial blend into autism mode as well.

The exposure of your child to any of these events needs to be carefully balanced against the risk of worsening the intestinal bacteria towards autism.

For instance, I would argue that most children require antibiotics for pneumonia but many do not for the runny nose that persists for 2 weeks.

And likewise, some vaccines are more critical than others. MMR protects against crippling, fatal illnesses while the chickenpox vaccine has much less of an impact on survival.

I think virtually all children will benefit from my protocol. It will protect those with mild bacterial imbalance from developing a mild developmental issue or developing ADD, headaches or depression later on in childhood.

And since it is proving effective enough to reverse some of the features of autism, it may be strong enough to lessen the risk of developing autism in those children with a more severe bacterial imbalance.

Obviously, the issue whether or not to vaccinate your child should not be taken lightly. I recommend discussing these issues with your physician before deciding to avoid or delay vaccination.

8

RECOGNIZING AND MANAGING PROPIONIC ACID RELAPSE

M aintaining improved health in children, just like maintaining improved health in adults, may involve dealing with new injuries and bacterial overgrowth relapses.

As previously explained in this book, autism, developmental disorders and cumulative brain injury (ADD, hyperactivity, anxiety, headaches, etc.) all require uncontrolled inflammation and the priming of microglia from bacterial overgrowth of the small intestine.

And in the case of autism, because excessive amounts of propionic acid are such critical factors in the health of the children, this is my first line of inquiry when I hear about signs of relapse in my patients.

It has been my experience that as long as bacterial overgrowth is controlled with daily inulin or reversed with a short course of rifaximin, and as long as my patient's inflammation is down-regulated correctly with proper doses of omega-3 and omega-9 fatty acids with a simultaneous elimination of omega-6 fatty acids, the symptoms of autism, developmental disorders, and cumulative brain injury continue to slowly improve over time.

But on occasion, I have also seen instances of relapse occur when the symptoms of autism or cumulative brain injury return.

Relapses may occur when the level of propionic acids rises and/or the level of pro-inflammatory cytokines increase significantly.

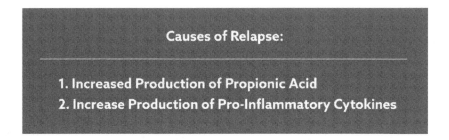

Causes of Relapse:

1. Increased Production of Propionic Acid
2. Increase Production of Pro-Inflammatory Cytokines

The good news is that those scenarios are sometimes preventable, they are often recognizable and just temporary in nature, and they often do not result in the significant loss of prior recovery if they are dealt with appropriately in a timely fashion.

This chapter of the book will deal expressly with management of symptomatic relapse due to propionic acid toxicity while issues involved with inflammatory relapse will be discussed in the following chapter.

PROPIONIC ACID RELAPSE OCCURS IN THOSE WITH PRIOR AUTISM DIAGNOSIS

The production of propionic acid is a process that cannot be completely turned off because the bacteria that normally reside within the colon naturally make propionic acid.

Therefore, it is not something that we can "fix" instead it is something we take efforts to "control" in that child. Therefore, there is always a risk of propionic acid toxicity if something disrupts the balance of intestinal bacteria.

Relapses from an increase in propionic acid occur when the bacterial overgrowth within the small intestine worsens and the bacteria begin secreting excessive amounts of propionic acid again.

The return of bacterial overgrowth is either permanent or temporary depending on the method of treatment that is used to control the overgrowth.

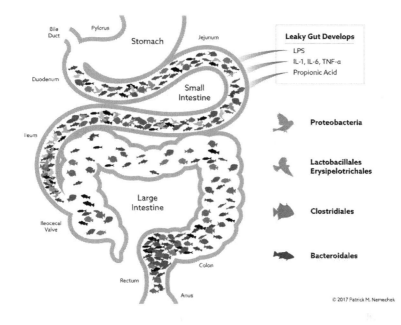

I believe that a relapse of bacterial overgrowth is temporary if the patient is being maintained on daily inulin supplementation because the inulin will continue to nourish the healthy bacteria, while those patients previously treated with rifaximin often experience a permanent relapse requiring retreatment in the same manner as before to sweep back the invading colonic bacteria.

Relapse from propionic acid toxicity generally only happens in children, teens, or young adults with prior autism.

As a rule, propionic acid relapse would not occur in individuals diagnosed with only developmental disorder or cumulative brain injuries and without a prior history of autism.

RECOGNIZING THE SYMPTOMS AND TIMING OF PROPIONIC ACID RELAPSE

It has been my experience that the symptoms of propionic acid relapse commonly occur within one to two weeks of the offending event to my patient's health.

Within this time frame, the child will exhibit decreased cognitive and neurological functioning as their propionic acid levels increase from their bacterial overgrowth.

The child will often exhibit the same patterns of impaired behavior (loss of eye-contact, disconnection from surroundings, suppressed energy levels, etc.) that they experienced before taking back control over their bacterial overgrowth with either inulin or rifaximin.

The two features that differentiate propionic acid relapse from an inflammatory relapse are (1) the speed of the onset of symptoms, and (2) the return of autistic behaviors.

Since bacterial overgrowth is required for the increase in propionic acid levels, there is often a triggering event for the bacterial overgrowth as well as a return of the child's intestinal symptoms.

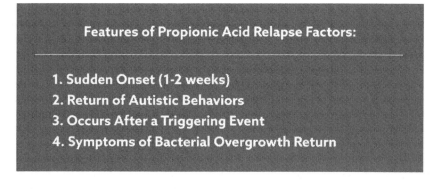

Features of Propionic Acid Relapse Factors:

1. Sudden Onset (1-2 weeks)
2. Return of Autistic Behaviors
3. Occurs After a Triggering Event
4. Symptoms of Bacterial Overgrowth Return

Since bacterial overgrowth is required for the increase in propionic acid levels, there is often a triggering event for the bacterial over-growth as well as a return of the child's intestinal symptoms.

Within a one to two-week time frame, propionic relapsing children will become much more subdued and withdrawn in their behavior.

My patient's families report that their children often seem to sleep more, they have less eye contact, they are less interactive, and they might be more moody, anxious, or angry.

Sometimes the symptoms of propionic acid may return in a mild form and for an afternoon they might resemble the behavior in any otherwise heathy child or adolescent who is just tired or in a bad mood that day.

The important point is that the symptoms of propionic relapse will persist for more than just an occasional afternoon.

In contrast, relapses from increased pro-inflammatory cytokine levels are subtle (less focus, worse concentration, more anxious, more fidgeting, increased hunger) and these changes may take longer for my patient's family to recognize.

Those subtle changes often occur a little later in time, over two to six weeks, before being recognized by a patient's family and they do not involve the child's prior autistic behaviors.

The symptoms of propionic acid relapse can only occur with the return of bacterial overgrowth; therefore, the onset of symptoms is often related to events that may result in the return of bacterial overgrowth.

The obvious triggering events for propionic acid relapse include the use of antibiotics, abdominal surgery, general anesthesia, an excessive or an adverse reaction to vaccination, potent antacid use, colonoscopy, intestinal infections (viral, bacterial or parasitic), severe food poisoning, or brain injury.

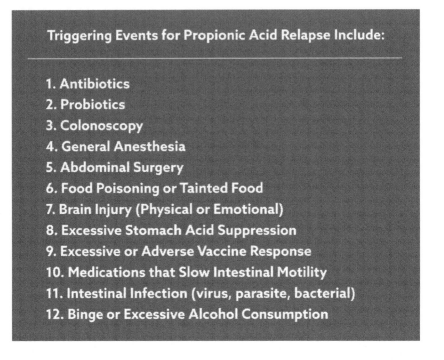

Triggering Events for Propionic Acid Relapse Include:

1. Antibiotics
2. Probiotics
3. Colonoscopy
4. General Anesthesia
5. Abdominal Surgery
6. Food Poisoning or Tainted Food
7. Brain Injury (Physical or Emotional)
8. Excessive Stomach Acid Suppression
9. Excessive or Adverse Vaccine Response
10. Medications that Slow Intestinal Motility
11. Intestinal Infection (virus, parasite, bacterial)
12. Binge or Excessive Alcohol Consumption

One not so obvious trigger, but one I mention as I am discussing my work with teenage and young adult patients, is binge alcohol drinking especially with alcoholic spirits (greater than 20% alcohol).

The acute neurotoxic effects of alcohol can slow down the movement of the digestive tract and can allow bacterial migration and bacterial overgrowth to resume.

While alcohol consumption may sound like an awkward subject to include in a book about childhood disorders, the reality of underage drinking and a youth or young adult's access to alcohol in the home or in social settings may someday be relevant to their health and their risk of bacterial overgrowth relapse.

If a propionic acid relapse occurs in my patient, I will consider retreating the bacterial overgrowth as I feel is necessary. However, continued inulin or repeated rifaximin alone is never sufficient treatment for my patients to maintain control over their bacterial overgrowth.

It is important for me to try to determine why my patient has had a propionic acid relapse. I will ask their parents if all of the other aspects of The Nemechek Protocol™ are being consistently followed or if other things (medications, vitamins, supplements, herbs, oils, teas, etc.) have been added or substituted that deviate from my Protocol.

Over the years I have heard many reasons why there was a lapse in 100% adherence to my Protocol, but there are simply no days off when it comes to maintaining improved health.

All too often I hear about a family vacation or a week away at camp when all or part of the patient's treatment (fish oil or inulin) was left behind at home. Laxity with compliance might occur during the celebration of holidays or when special occasions brought omega-6 foods back into the patient's diet.

I have also heard how once a routine was established, parental supervision relaxed and the parents relied on their teenager to remember to take their own fish oil.

Propionic acid production, in sharp contrast, never takes time off for a vacation or to go to camp. It does not observe holidays and it will not forget to produce excessive amounts whenever it is given an opportunity to do so.

The easiest aspect about what I do with my patients to control propionic acid toxicity, which is also the hardest aspect, is that the core tools in The Nemechek Protocol™ are so simple yet they require consistency, patience, and persistence.

For my patients to learn that daily fish oil and the elimination of omega-6 vegetable oils in the diet is mandatory to create the opportunity for the brain to move the intestinal tract more efficiently to resist propionic acid relapse is one thing, but to actually change each meal and to never forget a patient's daily dosage is quite another thing.

Many of my patient's parents have inquired about the high rate of spontaneous relapse of bacterial overgrowth after the use of rifaximin as reported in patients with irritable bowel syndrome (IBS).

Spontaneous relapse is often a consequence of slowed intestinal motility from autonomic nervous system dysfunction which is a fundamental aspect of the pathophysiology of IBS.

I have found that bacterial overgrowth relapse in children and adolescents is generally infrequent when rifaximin is used as part of The Nemechek Protocol™.

My patients using The Nemechek Protocol™ experience significant improvement of intestinal motility because my Protocol also helps reverse underlying autonomic nervous system dysfunction.

The reason for this distinction is because my patient's brains can more effectively move their digestive tract forward as a result of improved autonomic nervous system function.

The improvement of autonomic nervous system function is the reason why my treatment discovery is so different, and this is what defines the success of The Nemechek Protocol™ in children and adults alike.

IMPORTANT COMMENT REGARDING TRIGGERS OF RELAPSE:

I emphasize to my patients that the list of triggers is not a list of events to be avoided but are instead a list of events to be recognized as potential triggers in some people. They are not potential triggers of relapse in all people, or in all situations.

There are many situations in which a child's health and life is, or might be, endangered if they do not receive something that appears on that list such as take antibiotics, get a vaccine, or have a surgery.

I advocate that all of my patients receive the appropriate and/or preventative medical care that is necessary for them to achieve and maintain their health and safety.

It is important for parents to discuss the necessity of exposing their child to any potential trigger event with their physicians, as well as discussing the potential harmful consequences of not exposing their child to such an event, before making the decision that they deem is best for their child.

RECOGNIZING RELAPSE OF BACTERIAL OVERGROWTH

As a rule, I always note what intestinal issues improved in my patients after their use of rifaximin as a benchmark for me to determine if their symptoms from bacterial overgrowth have returned.

Once their bacterial overgrowth returns, my patient's intestinal function often worsens and parallels the intestinal and digestive issues they had experienced prior to starting The Nemechek Protocol™.

If my patient had constipation and abdominal cramps prior to being treated with rifaximin, those are the same symptoms that often will return.

Or if my patient had loose stools (diarrhea) and were intolerant to certain foods such as lettuce or bananas, those symptoms will also likely return.

Being mindful of intestinal function and digestive issues if children relapse allows their parents and their physicians to recognize the return of these symptoms and to treat the relapse appropriately with only a minimal amount of neurological regression.

And once properly retreated, I have seen that children are often quickly restored to their level of improved health.

DIFFERENCES IN PROPIONIC ACID RELAPSE BETWEEN INULIN-USING VS. RIFAXIMIN-TREATED PATIENTS

The main difference I have seen in propionic acid relapse between those children maintained on inulin and the children, adolescents, or adults who have been treated with rifaximin is in what needs to be done to restore control of bacterial overgrowth and suppress propionic acid production after a relapse.

My inulin-treated patients recover spontaneously after any of the above events as long as they continue their daily supplementation of prebiotic inulin fiber.

The inulin will not lose effectiveness, and the prior dosage of inulin is typically adequate to restore their bacterial control.

My patient may have a transient suppression or alteration in their neurological functioning as described in previous chapters from the increase in propionic acid but those issues typically recover within a week or so after the offending event resolves, is treated, or is completed.

If this does not help my patient, I have seen that a slight increase in their daily inulin dose usually improves the situation.

My patients who are children, adolescents, or adults who I have previously treated with rifaximin and who experience a propionic acid relapse will typically need to be retreated with rifaximin again.

The dosage of rifaximin that I use with a relapse is the same that I used initially to achieve their reversal of bacterial overgrowth.

Similar to my patients who are on continual treatment with inulin, the recovery from propionic acid toxicity after retreatment with rifaximin is rather rapid with the patient generally returning to their pre-event neurological baseline often within one to two weeks after completing the rifaximin.

In addition, re-treatment with rifaximin often has fewer side effects than what my patient might have experienced during their initial treatment.

I believe that fewer side effects during re-treatment may be due to their improved intestinal motility as a result of autonomic nervous system improvement.

And fortunately, unlike other types of antibiotics, retreatment with rifaximin does not seem to alter the overall blend of intestinal bacteria and the development of microbial resistance to rifaximin is a very rare phenomenon.

PROPIONIC ACID RELAPSE IN CHILDREN WHO HAVE OUTGROWN THE BENEFIT OF INULIN

I have previously mentioned my observations that my patients who are children around 10 to 13 years of age and adolescents may not respond as well to daily inulin suppression of bacterial overgrowth as children who are less than 10 years of age.

The scientific reasons for this are not clear but from a practical standpoint this is why I recommend rebalancing intestinal bacteria with rifaximin in my older patients who did not respond to inulin, and in all adolescents and adults.

The age threshold that appears to affect a patient's response to inulin begs the hypothetical question: "Could a child who has experienced a previously good response to inulin somewhat outgrow the therapeutic inulin prebiotic effect as they age and suffer a propionic relapse?".

In other words, if a child has had an excellent response with The Nemechek Protocol™ using inulin at the age of 8, might they experience a relapse at some point as they age into adolescence that is not controlled with inulin?

I believe this is possible, but as of yet, I have not had any continual young inulin patients in my practice who have outgrown the benefit of prebiotic inulin.

My guess is that if it happens it may present in the following manner: that a child will be well-controlled using inulin as part of The Nemechek Protocol™ and they will suffer a relapse from one of the common events previously mentioned.

But instead of simply recovering shortly after the relapse-triggering event resolves, the child does not recover or regain their improved health with continued inulin use.

If this were to happen, and no other supplements had been added and there has been complete compliance with all the other prongs of

The Nemechek Protocol™, then I anticipate I might treat the child with rifaximin at that point.

Pointer:

Watch for neurological changes more than stool changes.

When looking for signs of a propionic acid relapse in a patient, I am first and foremost looking for changes and regression in neurological function.

There seems to be a general over-focus on the frequency and quality of stool production of the children. If we were to examine every stool of an average adult every single day, they would not only feel overanalyzed, but we would observe a variety of stool changes that do not mean anything.

I tell my patients it is more important to watch for changes in brain function than it is to watch for changes in the bathroom.

Intestinal symptoms alone do not mean that excessive propionic acid production has resumed.

9

RECOGNIZING AND MANAGING INFLAMMATORY RELAPSE

M y first concern when I see the relapse of symptoms in a patient is whether or not a propionic acid relapse has occurred.

My second concern is whether the patient is experiencing an inflammatory relapse that is the source of their symptoms.

Causes of Relapse:

1. Increased Production of Propionic Acid
2. Increase Production of Pro-Inflammatory Cytokines

Like another increase of propionic acid production, another increase in pro-inflammatory cytokines is also sometimes preventable, is often easily recognizable and temporary in nature, and often does not result in significant loss of prior recovery if dealt with appropriately in a timely fashion.

This chapter will deal expressly with management of symptomatic relapse due to increased levels of pro-inflammatory cytokines.

Worsening of symptoms from the first cause of relapse from increased propionic acid toxicity was discussed in the preceding chapter.

THE EFFECT OF THE NEMECHEK PROTOCOL™ ON INFLAMMATION

From an inflammatory perspective, The Nemechek Protocol™ results in three major physiological shifts that allow neuronal pruning to increase development and the repair of cumulative brain injury to occur.

First, The Nemechek Protocol™ reduces the production of pro-inflammatory cytokines from both bacterial overgrowth and from an omega-6 to omega-3 fatty acid ratio imbalance in the patient's diet.

Second, The Nemechek Protocol™ reduces inflammatory stress caused by the excessive amounts of linoleic, arachidonic, and palmitic acids found in prepared and processed foods.

And third, The Nemechek Protocol™ shifts the activation state of the M1-microglia from their inflammatory and cytokine production behavior towards the anti-inflammatory M2-microglia which are associated with the release of anti-inflammatory cytokines (IL-10, TGF- β1) and the repair of injured brain cells.

Inflammatory Benefits of The Nemechek Protocol™:

1. Balances Omega-6 to Omega-3 Fatty Acids
2. Reduces the Impact of Dietary Linoleic, Arachidonic, and Palmitic Acids
3. Shifts M1-Microglia towards the Anti-inflammatory M2-Microglia Behavior

RECOGNIZING RELAPSE FROM INCREASED PRO-INFLAMMATORY CYTOKINE LEVELS

As previously discussed, a relapse from increased levels of propionic acid happens when the bacterial overgrowth within the small intestine reoccurs and the bacteria begin secreting excessive amounts of propionic acid again.

Propionic acid levels often increase rapidly and result in the rapid relapse of propionic acid behaviors.

The return of symptoms from an inflammatory relapse that I have seen in my patients, however, is distinctly different.

The most important difference is that inflammatory relapse occurs more slowly, often over a two to six-week timeframe, unlike propionic acid relapse which occurs rapidly in just one to two weeks.

The characteristic nature of inflammatory relapse is related to the symptoms of the patient's underlying autonomic nervous system dysfunction that had been improving, and is not necessarily related to the symptoms of propionic acid toxicity.

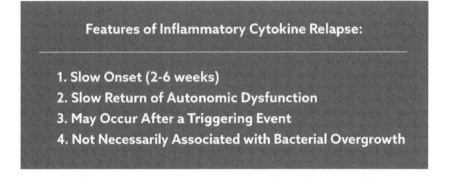

Features of Inflammatory Cytokine Relapse:

1. Slow Onset (2-6 weeks)
2. Slow Return of Autonomic Dysfunction
3. May Occur After a Triggering Event
4. Not Necessarily Associated with Bacterial Overgrowth

The triggers of inflammatory relapses are events that cause an increase in pro-inflammatory cytokine levels within the brain.

The pro-inflammatory cytokines most commonly linked to deteriorating neurological function are IL-2, IL-6 and TNF-alpha.

These cytokines are released from the "leaky gut" phenomenon that occurs with bacterial overgrowth.

But unlike clinical relapse from propionic acid toxicity, a worsening of symptoms from an increase in pro-inflammatory cytokines does not necessarily require bacterial overgrowth.

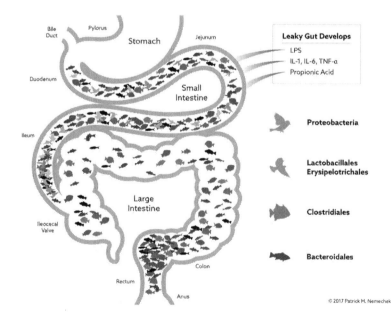

Although bacterial overgrowth can contribute to both propionic acid relapse as well as inflammatory relapse, the source of pro-inflammatory cytokines causing an inflammatory relapse can come from a variety of sources (discussed below) both within and outside of the central nervous system.

Some of the triggering events are short-lived and their adverse effects are transient as long as the patient continues to adhere to The Nemechek Protocol™.

Examples of short term inflammatory triggers are fractures, acute infectious states (sinusitis, urinary tract infection), stress from abdominal or thoracic surgery, excessive or adverse reactions to vaccinations, and other infections.

Short Term Inflammatory Relapse Events:

1. Fractures
2. Pneumonia
3. Viral Infection
4. Urinary Tract Infections
5. Sinus/Middle Ear Infection
6. Abdominal or Thoracic Surgery
7. Excessive or Adverse Vaccination Reactions

Other types of events may lead to the long term production of increased levels of pro-inflammatory cytokines.

Examples of events that may fuel a patient's rise in pro-inflammatory cytokines includes the increased inflammation that results from the return of intestinal bacterial overgrowth, the non-adherence to their daily dosing of inulin (if applicable), from switching to a low-quality fish oil or olive oil that no longer protects or repairs the cells and the development of an autoimmune disorder (Hashimoto's, Crohn's, Psoriasis).

In addition, chronic exposure to second-hand tobacco smoke or diesel fumes, severe vitamin D deficiency, periodontal disease, and chronic infections (hepatitis, HIV, intestinal parasite) can also contribute to long term relapse.

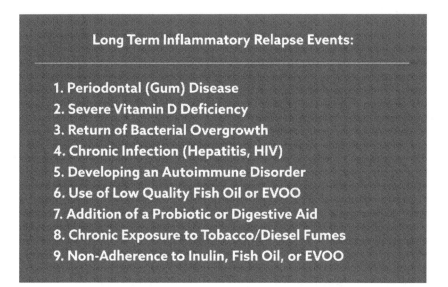

Long Term Inflammatory Relapse Events:

1. Periodontal (Gum) Disease
2. Severe Vitamin D Deficiency
3. Return of Bacterial Overgrowth
4. Chronic Infection (Hepatitis, HIV)
5. Developing an Autoimmune Disorder
6. Use of Low Quality Fish Oil or EVOO
7. Addition of a Probiotic or Digestive Aid
8. Chronic Exposure to Tobacco/Diesel Fumes
9. Non-Adherence to Inulin, Fish Oil, or EVOO

The worsening of symptoms from increased pro-inflammatory cytokines can occur in any patient that is recovering from a developmental disorder or who has residual brain damage (autonomic nervous system dysfunction, chronic depression, PTSD) from prior physical, emotional or inflammatory brain injuries (cumulative brain injury).

SYMPTOMS OF RELAPSE FROM INCREASED INFLAMMATION

The symptoms that children experience can be categorized as belonging to propionic acid toxicity, developmental delay, and cumulative brain injury.

The symptoms I see in my patients from propionic acid toxicity are the regressive, sedate behaviors often reported by their parents shortly after a classic regressive episode (loss of eye contact, fatigue, repetitive behaviors, altered appetite).

The symptoms I see in my patients associated with developmental delay involve inadequate neuronal development leading to sensory, speech, or motor difficulties.

And the symptoms I see in my patients that are associated with cumulative brain injury (CBI), are often involved with the dysfunction of their autonomic nervous system but may also involve regions of their brain dealing with emotional and vestibular function.

PPA Toxicity	Developmental Delay	CBI
Loss of Eye Contact	Sensory Processing Disorder	Anxiety, Stimming
Self-Isolation	Motor-Gait Dysfunction	Increased Hunger
Fatigue	Delayed of Impaired Speech	ADD, ADHD, PTSD
Limited Food Preference		Hyperactivity
Repetitive Behaviors		Bladder Issues
		Chronic Depression

Interestingly, when I see patients experience a purely inflammatory relapse (meaning there is no bacterial overgrowth and no increase in propionic acid), the symptoms that worsen tend to be from those symptoms associated with cumulative brain injury and not symptoms reflective of their prior developmental issues.

In my patients with developmental delay, the symptomatic improvement associated with renewed neuronal pruning is seen in their renewed brain maturation after they start working with me on The Nemechek Protocol™.

Children and adolescents will start moving forward from a neurological-developmental standpoint. Their emotional, social, sensory, and physical function begins to catch up to their chronological age.

And perhaps the single most inspiring thing about the brain repair process that I see happening in my patients is that once their neuronal pruning and maturation has occurred it generally cannot be reversed (in other words, the new neuronal pathways are not "unpruned") with an inflammatory relapse.

If my patients have overcome developmental delay and they have learned certain social skills, or they have learned how to speak more clearly, the patients generally do not experience a deterioration of their prior developmental gains with an inflammatory relapse.

Not only do these children not deteriorate to the point where we first began the repair process, their families now better understand the repair process and that ongoing repair is still underway.

The symptoms predominantly associated with an inflammatory relapse are those related to the underlying cumulative brain injury that is still in the process of being repaired.

To use an old adage, inflammatory relapse amounts to a "3-steps forward, 1-step backwards" scenario consisting mainly of gradual gains (forward) with potential relapses of cumulative brain injury (backwards) after a short term or a long term inflammatory relapse event.

The repair of autonomic nervous system damage from cumulative brain injury is seen in the reduction of hyperactivity, excessive hunger, unprovoked anxiety or aggression, stimming, toe-walking, chronic fatigue, as well as improved focus and attention.

During an inflammatory relapse, it is the symptoms of autonomic nervous system dysfunction that slowly return over several weeks if the patient's inflammatory cytokine levels remain chronically elevated.

For example, if my patient has improvement in their level of hyperactivity, anxiety, and excessive hunger while on The Nemechek Protocol™ and then for some reason their supplementation with fish oil was stopped or switched to a brand that is lower quality or fraudulent, their inflammatory cytokines may surge.

In that example, the drop or the lack of the core omega-3 nutrients in the fish oil results in a steady and chronic elevation of pro-inflammatory cytokines within the brain, and over the next two to six weeks there would be a gradual return of the child's hyperactivity, anxiety, and excessive hunger.

Therefore, in order for me to recognize the signs and symptoms of any type of relapse in my patients, I first think of the symptoms of (1) propionic acid toxicity, (2) developmental delay, and (3) cumulative brain injury as three different problems with distinct timelines and symptoms that are unique to each brain process that may be involved.

SOMETIMES RELAPSE DOES NOT MAKE SENSE

Even as a skilled clinician, sometimes there are clinical scenarios where I cannot sort out if my patient is experiencing a propionic acid relapse requiring another round of rifaximin or a simple inflammatory relapse that might just require a boost in their fish oil dosage.

The first thing I do is to double check that no probiotics have been added back in to my patient's supplements or foods. While I understand how some patients with bacterial overgrowth have had some positive benefit from probiotics in the past, once their overgrowth has been reversed with inulin or rifaximin I have observed the same probiotic to significantly worsen my patient's condition.

The second thing that I do is to review their history to see if any new diets, medications, or supplements have been added at the same time they are on The Nemechek Protocol™ or if a dosage was changed without my approval. Sometimes unexpected side effects from these other types of things can mimic propionic acid or inflammatory relapses.

If something new was added or if a doses were changed, I consider having the family stop the diet, medication, supplement, or go back to the previous dosage to see if the symptoms will resolve.

And finally, if the symptoms do not improve after several weeks and if none of the above issues apply to the patient, I will often simply just rebalance the intestinal tract with another course of rifaximin or I potentially would consider making the shift from inulin to rifaximin.

Following this step-by-step approach usually helps me solve the mystery of unexplained inflammatory relapses.

CAUTION:

Do not ever stop any prescription medication or alter the dosage without first discussing all of the potential risks with the prescribing physician.

10

POTENTIAL OPPORTUNITIES FOR PREVENTION

Now that I have discovered a process that can reverse or improve key features in existing autism and many other childhood disorders, I naturally consider whether this same process may be used in a potentially preventative manner.

If I can make a change in the children of today, what about making a change in the children of tomorrow?

The reduction of inflammation and bacterial overgrowth may be the key elements in preventing many childhood developmental disorders.

In the case of autism, the first challenge is whether we can prevent the excessive production of propionic acid from bacterial overgrowth as it the unique pathological feature that delineates most autism from other disorders.

If we can maintain a healthier balance of intestinal bacteria in a child without overgrowth and without the excessive production of propionic acid, the main features that delineate autism from developmental delay and cumulative brain injury would predictably not occur.

A healthier balance of intestinal bacteria would also predictably prevent the leakage of lipopolysaccharide (LPS) into the systemic circulation and central nervous system.

Prevention of LPS leakage (also known as bacterial translocation or leaky gut) might also prevent two additional pathological events from occurring:

1. Production of pro-inflammatory cytokines from the small intestine
2. Development of inflammation-promoting, primed M1-microglia (white blood cells within the CNS)

Pro-inflammatory cytokines and primed M1-microglia only serve to slow normal neuronal pruning (a causative factor in developmental delay) as well as magnify the damage and prevent full recovery from common childhood brain injuries.

In this chapter, I have included the recommendations I discuss with my patients that address potential methods to limit or reduce the risk of a child from developing clinically harmful overgrowth of intestinal bacterial, and consequently limit the risk of developing autism, developmental delay, and cumulative brain injury.

None of my possible prevention suggestions in this chapter are "proven" in the sense that human clinical trials have been performed.

My theories come from my experiences and observations after treating adults of all ages, children with autism and developmental disorders, and women before and after pregnancy with The Nemechek Protocol™.

All of these patients were suffering from ill-effects from inflammation, bacterial overgrowth, and autonomic nervous system dysfunction.

I have been able to reverse or greatly improve the bacterial overgrowth in mothers of child-bearing age and children of all ages so there is reasonable potential that the same methods that prevent bacterial overgrowth might also prevent or limit the development of autism as well as developmental delay and cumulative brain injury since they are commonly the consequence of bacterial overgrowth.

And since these childhood disorders are very diverse in nature, as can be some of the complicating factors that arise during pregnancy.

Any readers of this book who are learning about the treatment modalities and suggestions that I give to my patients must fully discuss any and all of these potential treatment modalities and suggestions with their healthcare providers before initiating any of them with any person, or at any time either prior to pregnancy, during pregnancy, or after delivery.

The failure of anyone to inform all of their managing physicians of all of their medications, supplements, herbs, intention to follow any treatment program, dietary habits, etc., may confuse the clinical picture for their physicians and even cause unnecessary medication use, side effects, or complications.

CONSIDERATIONS BEFORE PREGNANCY

Women considering pregnancy need to be aware that pro-inflammatory cytokines (IL-1, IL-6, TNF-alpha) that are produced within their body are capable of crossing the placenta and causing potential harm to their unborn child.

Pro-inflammatory cytokines are capable of disrupting normal brain development as well as activating genes in their child while still within the womb and after birth.

After birth, they may even be capable of causing new mutations within the child's DNA. These cytokines are also associated with increased pregnancy complications such as miscarriage and eclampsia.

I advise my female patients who are considering becoming pregnant to work towards normalizing their body's inflammatory status. The Nemechek Protocol™ for Autonomic Recovery (for adults) is designed to specifically reduce a person's excessive levels of pro-inflammatory cytokines in order to improve or restore autonomic nervous system dysfunction.

Waiting until a woman becomes pregnant before starting the process of general inflammation reduction is not a good strategy because it may take three or more months to achieve a lower or normal state of inflammatory cytokines.

Likewise, waiting until a woman becomes pregnant before starting the process of bacterial overgrowth management is also not a good strategy because prebiotic inulin supplementation takes time to work.

The rifaximin medication I prescribe to my adult patients to reverse intestinal bacterial overgrowth is not a treatment option as it is not approved for use during pregnancy or breastfeeding.

The reduction of overall inflammation prior to pregnancy may improve fertility rates and may possibly limit complications such as pre-eclampsia and miscarriage during pregnancy.

Inflammation reduction may also improve the mother's autonomic nervous system health and resilience against the strain and potential injury that is sometimes caused during delivery.

I believe that insuring a woman does not have significant bacterial overgrowth and supplementing their diet with the correct balance of omega-3 and omega-6 fatty acids via The Nemechek Protocol™ will go a long way towards maximizing their chances for a healthy and uncomplicated pregnancy.

CONSIDERATIONS DURING PREGNANCY

Inflammation can play a role in affecting the child's neurological development prior to birth while they are still developing within the womb.

Excessive exposure of the fetus to elevated levels of pro-inflammatory cytokines is an important contributing factor that might also determine the presence or the level of severity of autism or other developmental disorders at the time of birth.

Sources of pro-inflammatory cytokine exposure during pregnancy may include intestinal bacterial imbalance of the mother, inadequate omega-3 and excessive omega-6 fatty acids dietary intakes, exposure to tobacco smoke, periodontal disease, excessive dietary AGEs (advanced glycation end products) intake as well as maternal dysfunction of the parasympathetic-vagus inflammatory reflex of the autonomic nervous system.

After the birth of a child, excessive pro-inflammatory cytokines can cause disruption of the normal process of neuronal development and inhibit the brain from repairing commonplace brain injuries that occur from physical, emotional, chemical, and inflammatory trauma.

Bacterial Colonization versus Bacterial Translocation During Pregnancy

The developing fetus does not have any bacteria within their intestines while they are in the womb so they cannot develop inflammation from bacterial translocation before birth.

The child's intestinal tract becomes colonized with their mother's bacterial blend at the time of birth, so the child inherits the mother's bacterial blend.

Recent studies suggest that the child will adopt the mother's intestinal bacterial blend regardless if the delivery is a vaginal birth or by a caesarian section.

If the mother has a healthy blend of intestinal bacteria, the child is colonized with a healthy blend at birth.

The excessive inflammation from intestinal bacteria in a child may increase immediately after birth if they are colonized with an unhealthy blend of intestinal bacteria they adopt from their mother, or if their blend is disrupted by spending time within the NICU or by receiving antibiotics.

If mother has a blend that is prone to bacterial overgrowth, inflammation, and propionic acid production then the child will similarly be born with bacterial overgrowth, inflammation, and the propensity to produce propionic acid.

LPS (lipopolysaccharide) is a molecule from the surface of over-growth bacteria that leaks across the intestine and triggers inflammation in a process known as bacterial translocation (often referred to as leaky gut).

Animal studies indicate that bacterial translocation of LPS in the mother does not trigger inflammation in the fetus but it will trigger an increase of pro-inflammatory cytokines within the mother.

Unfortunately, these cytokines are able to cross the placenta and alter the child's neurological development as well as trigger the variety of genes that add to the complexity of autism (ASD) and intrauterine developmental disorders.

Improving Omega-3 Fatty Acid Transfer in the Third Trimester

The mother will transfer half of her entire bodily omega-3 reserves to her child during the third trimester of pregnancy.

This transfer provides the child with enough omega-3 fatty acids required for normal neurological development during their first year of life.

The neurological improvement is so significant that the child of a mother supplementing with omega-3 fatty acids from fish oil on average will have an I.Q. that is almost 10 points higher than they would have had otherwise.

But if the mother's diet is low in omega-3 fatty acids and high in inflammation causing omega-6 fatty acids, the child may experience a similar imbalance of omega fatty acids during the third trimester transfer.

The omega fatty acid imbalance will further increase the inflammatory cytokine level within the mother and child and may further impair normal brain development in the child.

Supplementation with extra virgin olive oil can also help reduce the inflammatory state of the mother even further during pregnancy. Extra virgin olive oil contains high amounts of an omega-9 fatty acid called oleic acid.

Oleic acid helps block and reverse the inflammatory damaged caused by excessive dietary omega-6 fatty acid intake, as well as saturated fatty acids such as palmitic acid.

I typically recommend that the expectant mothers under my care supplement with 2,000-3,000 mg of fish oil per day, and that they also consume 2 tablespoons of domestic, certified extra virgin olive oil.

Many regions of the world produce excellent, high quality olive oil locally which is an ideal choice to cook with but because of the high percentage of fraudulent olive oil being imported into the U.S., I recommend that my U.S. patients consume only California Olive Oil Council (COOC) certified olive oils from California because of their high quality.

Improving Intestinal Bacterial Balance During Pregnancy

To improve intestinal balance during pregnancy, I recommend my patients supplement if needed with the over the counter prebiotic fiber inulin.

Inulin helps improve the intestinal symptoms of bacterial overgrowth such as diarrhea, heartburn, nausea, and cramping.

Unfortunately, intestinal balance treatment options during pregnancy are limited to just the inulin fiber.

The use of the non-absorbable antibiotic rifaximin to rebalance the intestinal bacteria has not been adequately studied during pregnancy, and cannot be recommended for use during pregnancy.

CONSIDERATIONS AFTER BIRTH

Maximizing a healthy balance of intestinal bacteria along with maintaining a healthy balance between omega-3 and omega-6 fatty acids is critical for normal brain development and normal neuronal repair of brain injuries that can commonly occur throughout life. Since reversing intestinal imbalance and restoring the omega-3 to omega-6 fatty acid balance reverses many of the key features in autism, managing these issues upfront may theoretically help prevent regressive autism from occurring in some children.

If there is any suspicion of bacterial overgrowth in the mother or older siblings (since they would also be colonized with the mother's bacterial blend of my patient, the younger sibling), I generally recommend supplementing the infant with 1/16 to 1/8 tsp of powdered inulin fiber daily and 300 mg of omega-3 fatty acids from fish oil.

When the child is old enough to eat regular food, I recommend that their food be cooked in certified California extra virgin olive oil to protect them from toxic omega-6 fatty acids that will inevitably seep into their diet.

CONSIDERATIONS SPECIFIC TO VACCINATIONS

Personally, I support the vaccination of children.

I am only against vaccinating children *when* they are experiencing bacterial overgrowth and *when* they have an unhealthy level of pro-inflammatory cytokines within their brain.

As I have discussed in previous chapters, the brain can be injured through physical injury, emotional traumas, by chemical or toxic exposures, by the lack of oxygen, and though a surge of inflammatory chemicals called pro-inflammatory cytokines.

These pro-inflammatory cytokines are part of our natural repair process. For instance, these chemicals are released with a healthy immune reaction triggered by influenza, and cause the fatigue and muscle discomfort we commonly experience.

These pro-inflammatory cytokines can be released under other common circumstances as well.

In animal studies surgeries of the abdomen or chest, fractures of the long bones, brain infections, and vaccines are all capable of disrupting brain function due to a release of pro-inflammatory cytokines.

It is important to note that when the pro-inflammatory cytokines injure the brain of a healthy mouse with a normal intestinal bacterial balance and normal omega fatty acid intakes, the mouse is capable of fully recovering from the inflammatory stress of the vaccine within a few weeks.

If a mouse has primed-microglia and increased levels of pro-inflammatory cytokines from bacterial overgrowth, the mouse does not fully recover and the injury leaves residual damage behind (see Cunningham papers in reference appendix).

The residual damage from unrepaired brain injury contributes to the cumulative brain injury that I have discussed elsewhere in this book.

Vaccinations are designed to mimic exposure to an infectious organism in order to create a protective inflammatory, immune reaction.

For a vaccine to be effective, the inflammation it triggers is an essential part of the protective reaction.

But depending on the brain health of the person vaccinated, the inflammatory surge of pro-inflammatory cytokines from the vaccine may have unintended consequences such as the worsening of bacterial overgrowth, developmental delay, or may result in cumulative brain damage.

Knowing that autism and the associated developmental delay cannot generally occur without the elevated propionic acid levels and inflammation triggered by bacterial overgrowth of the small intestine, the unavoidable question becomes how might the inflammatory reaction from the vaccine increase the likelihood of autism, developmental disorders or cumulative brain injury?

The debate has raged for decades over the direct and indirect consequences of vaccinations on the incidence of autism in particular.

My personal views of the possible role of vaccines in triggering autism is as follows:

The inflammatory surge commonly delivered by vaccines may be strong enough to even temporarily disrupt function of the autonomic nervous system and result in slowing of forward intestinal motility (peristalsis) in susceptible individuals.

Studies demonstrate that vaccines are capable of impairing the function of the parasympathetic branch of the autonomic nervous system.

Impaired parasympathetic function is associated with slowed peristalsis, a risk factor for the development or worsening of bacterial overgrowth.

Slowing of intestinal peristalsis from other situations such as general anesthesia, abdominal surgery, concussions, and disorders such as scleroderma and renal failure are all associated with an increased risk in the development of bacterial overgrowth of the small intestine.

In my office, I have witnessed the relapse of bacterial overgrowth from routine vaccination in several adult patients under my care.

If a child acquires a mild form of bacterial overgrowth from their mother or from the use of antibiotics early in the course of their life, a subsequent vaccination might worsen bacterial overgrowth and might encourage the excessive production of propionic acid though its negative effect on peristalsis.

In individuals with previously primed microglia from bacterial overgrowth, the added inflammatory surge could further slow development and could contribute a small amount of cumulative brain injury since the primed-microglia have been shown to prevent full recovery from vaccine-related brain injury.

Again, personally, I support the vaccination of children.

I am only against vaccinating children when they are experiencing bacterial overgrowth and when they have an unhealthy level of pro-inflammatory cytokines within their brain.

The issues then become when does a patient receive life-saving vaccinations that are necessary, and how might we improve the patient's health before and during such vaccinations.

Vaccines are the only way to presently protect children from several deadly illnesses for which there is no other treatment.

Vaccinations against measles and many other childhood illnesses have been a great success, and without vaccinations massive epidemics will once again become the deadly norm.

As a general health reminder, there are no antibiotics to treat a child infected with measles, mumps, rubella, or polio.

I feel that another important issue is the timing of the vaccinations.

I believe that delaying the vaccination of children for a few months until their intestinal bacteria and inflammatory status has been improved with inulin and omega-3 fatty acids from fish oil would predictably help their nervous systems to stabilize and should help to minimize the risk of developing autism, future developmental delay, and cumulative brain injury.

To explore possible preventative opportunities, I logically begin with the simple nutritional tools that impact existing autism and childhood disorders and I use them proactively by starting my infant or young child patient on daily inulin and fish oil supplementation.

Balancing the intestinal bacteria with 1/16 to 1/4 teaspoon of powdered inulin per day in my patient with suspected bacterial overgrowth has the potential to lessen the likelihood of bacterial overgrowth with propionic acid-producing bacteria from decreased peristalsis.

It is the sudden production of excessive and high levels of propionic acid from the intestinal tract that saturate the child's brain and explain why some parents report that they witnessed their child appear to drift away in a stuporous state shortly after receiving a vaccine.

Excessive propionic acid production is the cause of the classic regressive autism scenario.

In addition, supplementing with 300-500 mg of omega-3 fatty acids from fish oil and cooking all foods in certified California extra virgin oil olive should also help shift the phenotype of the microglia within the child's brain into the m2-microglia phenotype that are anti-inflammatory and help repair brain injuries.

And if my patient is consuming any form of processed food, I suggest adding a tiny amount of domestic, certified extra virgin olive oil to their daily diet to block the damaging effects of excessive omega-6 fatty acids.

Increasing the preponderance of repairing and anti-inflammatory M2-microglia should allow the child's brain to fully recover from any resulting inflammatory brain injury from the vaccine.

Balancing the need for vaccinations with the need to recover from intestinal bacterial overgrowth and inflammatory injury, brings us to the second timing issue which is the potential timeframe between rounds of vaccinations.

The possible timing manner in which I would approach the vaccinations in children suspected of experiencing bacterial overgrowth and/or an unhealthy level of pro-inflammatory cytokines within their brains would be to first start my young patient on daily inulin, fish oil supplementation. If they are consuming processed foods, I would also advise the addition of a tiny amount of domestic, certified olive oil to block the effects of excessive omega-6 fatty acids.

Then, after roughly three months, I would expect that the inflammation and microglial function should be improved adequately enough from the inulin and fish oil to begin vaccination with a single vaccine every 1 to 2 months in order to minimize the inflammatory surge of each exposure.

I keep in mind that the inflammatory surge that is expected after just one vaccine is significant. I would also think that receiving three vaccines in a single day would be expected to result in the cumulative effect of three separate inflammatory surges.

The MMR (measles, mumps and rubella) vaccine, for example, would ideally be split into a measles vaccination, then a mumps vaccination, and finally a rubella vaccine with each separated from the other by 1 to 2 months depending on that patient's individual rate of recovery.

It seems logical to me, when allowing recovery and stabilization time between rounds, that I might continue on like this with a single vaccine every month or two until a fully protective panel of vaccinations has been administered.

I readily admit that there are no "placebo-blinded human studies" to support my preventative recommendations contained in this chapter.

My recommendations come from deductive reasoning and common sense that if inulin and fish oil are able to reverse the neurological damage underlying autism and developmental delay, then the same treatments stand a reasonable chance of preventing them as well.

I do not anticipate human studies to be performed, or for peer-reviewed articles to be written anytime soon, on the beneficial effects of The Nemechek Protocol™.

But the reality we now face on a global level is that we suddenly have one or two generations of children who are experiencing increasing rates of autism and developmental disorders which until recently have been unexplained.

These children and others yet to be born need help, and I believe from the success I have seen using the simple nutritional tools of The Nemechek Protocol™ that this may be a possible preventative approach to be considered in the future as well.

As a reminder, none of my possible prevention suggestions in this chapter are "proven" in the sense that human clinical trials have been performed.

My theories come from my experiences and observations after treating adults of all ages, children with autism and developmental disorders, and women before and after pregnancy with The Nemechek Protocol™.

All of these patients were suffering from ill-effects from inflammation, bacterial overgrowth, and autonomic nervous system dysfunction.

11

SOMETIMES MIRACLES DO HAPPEN

STORIES OF RECOVERY

7-YEAR OLD BOY WITH DEVELOPMENTAL DELAY AND OPPOSITIONAL DEFIANCE DISORDER

This seven-year-old boy was brought to see me because behavioral and focus problems had deteriorated so much that his elementary school was trying to prevent him from entering 3rd grade.

He was having substantial trouble with focusing, he was easily distracted, he was excessively talkative, and he was very argumentative.

He had eczema, experienced frequent abdominal pain, would have random fevers, and he was a very picky eater. Two years earlier he had suffered a concussion after falling off of a trampoline.

He was started on inulin and omega-3 fatty acids from fish oil, and after only ten days his mother reported his eczema was dramatically improved and he was beginning to calm down.

After six weeks, his school performance and behavior had shown significant improvement. He was still struggling with some social interaction skills at this point.

After five months, behavioral problems were no longer being

reported by the school and the improvements in his academic performance ranked him near the top of his class.

After three years, he continues to do well as long as he continues on his inulin and fish oil supplementation.

5-YEAR OLD GIRL WITH NON-VERBAL AUTISM

This five-year-old girl had an uncomplicated birth but the mother felt her daughter had subtle behavioral issues from the very start.

She was showing substantial delay by six months of age. By this time, she already had received several courses of antibiotics for ear infections. After taking the antibiotics she developed severe eczema over her hands and face (a sign of intestinal bacterial imbalance).

At nine months of age she underwent cleft palate repair which resulted in a marked decrease in her overall functioning. She also developed acid reflux and eosinophilic esophagitis.

By age five she was having multiple problems and always seemed hungry and grumpy. She did not smile.

After six weeks of only being treated on inulin she tolerated the transition back to school without her usually emotional meltdowns that had often accompanied changes in her routine. The eczema on her skin had improved but she still had increased levels of hunger.

Fish oil was then added to her regimen and over the following 4 months her emotionality and learning skills greatly improved. Her eczema had disappeared and her hunger seemed to be reduced to a normal level.

She was beginning to speak clearly and she seemed to be picking up a few new words every week.

After one year of therapy, she was academically and emotionally functioning normally for her age. She still had occasional speech issues but for the most part she was fully conversational.

Three years later my wife and I bumped into this family at a local hardware store. She was running around and playing with her siblings in the aisles. Her mother said her daughter was "totally fine" and she was not having any issues that anyone could detect.

And we saw her smile.

23-YEAR OLD NON-VERBAL, AUTISTIC FEMALE WITH LENNOX-GASTAUT SYNDROME

I have seen the amazing potential for recovery in the adult autistic brain if provided the time necessary to heal as well as a consistent, persistent effort in maintaining The Nemechek Protocol™. I have mentioned this patient several times already but a more detailed explanation of her continued strides, all previously thought to be impossible to achieve, have given Jean and I great hope for all the other autistic children out there.

I first met her, a 23-year-old non-verbal autistic female with Lennox-Gastaut Syndrome, in 2015. This is a type of epilepsy with stiff or drop-type seizures.

There were minor complications that required her to be in the NICU for several days after her birth. By the age of ten months of age, she had begun having infantile spasms.

She never really learned to speak except a few words here and there, and developmentally her mother says things just seemed to worsen after the age of four. She was virtually unable to communicate.

When I first met her, she was having six to eight seizures per day in spite of being on multiple medications to stop the seizures. Due to the frequency and violent severity of these seizures her parents could never leave her unattended in a room by herself. She had ultimately given the diagnosis of Lennox-Gastaut Syndrome.

At the age of 23-years-old she had never held her parents gaze, she did not like to be held, she could not color or write, and she sat curled up in a chair most of the day rocking.

Her speech was limited to occasionally saying the name Michael which her parents believed to be an imaginary friend.

I initiated my Protocol of rifaximin for 10 days, high doses of omega-3 fatty acids, and I had her mother start cooking with California extra virgin olive oil.

Within eight weeks her seizures had dropped from six to eight per day, down to one or two seizures per day. The drop in her seizures was so significant her parents were able to start leaving her in a room by herself for short periods of time without fear that she would have a seizure that might hurt her. She would now sit upright in a chair and for the first time ever she slept through the night.

After four months of treatment, she started looking at her parents in the eyes. She began touching their cheeks and lips as if she was seeing them for the first time. She also wanted to be held, touched, and hugged as well.

At her six-month office visit, she started to smile at me and her seizures had reduced to one or two per week. We discovered she could now write her first name and last initial (although she had never been taught how to write) and she could draw objects that were recognizable.

After eight months, she began speaking rudimentary Spanish and English (she lived in a dual language household) but emotionally was behaving as if she were a three-year-old. She was having full tantrums in the grocery stores.

This was a difficult period for her parents because she was a grown woman who grabbed items off the shelves then would lay on the floor in the store crying over some item she wanted but that she could not have.

To get through it her parents just started buying those items and returning them to the store at a later time.

At her eighteenth-month office visit, she could speak very clearly in full sentences and her seizures had declined to one or two per month (despite the discontinuation of two out of her four seizure medications).

She spent a large part of her day playing dress up with clothes and shoes, and her mother gauged her emotional maturity to be about that of a five or six-year-old child.

At her twenty-seventh month visit she continues on her high dose of omega-3 fatty acids from fish oil and her mother is still cooking with olive oil.

I anticipate she may have relapses of her intestinal bacterial over-growth in the future and I plan to retreat her with rifaximin should that occur.

12

HOPE IS ON THE HORIZON

My patient example of a 23-year-old non-verbal autistic female with Lennox-Gastaut Syndrome teaches us that no matter how severe the autism, and no matter how significantly the developmental delay has slowed down brain maturation, the potential for improvement and recovery remains possible.

The human brain has an enormous capacity for repair and rejuvenation. The microglia within the brain are proving to be capable of restarting their task of synaptic-neuronal pruning even after many years of being in a state of inflammatory paralysis.

The substantial reduction of pro-inflammatory cytokines within the brain is all that is necessary for the normal process of maturation and brain repair to begin anew.

We are also beginning to understand that once human genes are turned on by inflammation, they can ultimately be shut off again once the inflammatory environment within the body is significantly reduced.

I gave this woman and her family the same advice I give to all my patients. To do their best to be patient, to give The Nemechek Protocol ™ and my overall approach to lower metabolic inflammation a chance, and to adopt a marathon mindset because brain recovery takes time and effort.

And because the path to recovery over all things medical is often five steps forward, and then sometimes one or two steps backwards, we compare today's behavior to a child's behavior that was months or years earlier.

Comparing today to yesterday will only serve to put parents on an emotional roller coaster, and it could possibly could lead parents to make some incorrect decisions for their child.

The neurons within the human brain, like the growing of your hair, can only grow and change so fast.

Every month, a child's brain can catch-up two to three months in development. That means for every calendar year, a recovering child may catch-up by two or three years.

I believe once the inflammation is suppressed, all that is required for continued recovery is a good solid inflammation suppressing regimen and patience.

Remember, the neurons within the human brain, like your hair, grow slowly and therefore your child's improvement will occur slowly but steadily.

APPENDIX I - AUTONOMIC DYSFUNCTION

MODERN DISEASE IS AUTONOMIC NERVOUS SYSTEM DYSFUNCTION

Understanding whether you have autonomic nervous system dysfunction is often the key to many of your medical mysteries.

The reversal of a wide range of symptoms, illnesses, and chronic diseases by repairing your cellular, brain, and nervous system damage is a new and whole-body approach to medicine. To fix the body, we must fix the brain.

Modern illness often begins with subtle changes in how our brain is able to coordinate and regulate our body. When our autonomic nervous system begins to malfunction we get headaches, heartburn, feel lightheaded or dizzy, anxious, have abnormal heart rhythms, or intestinal trouble. We may to go to the bathroom more often, experience chronic pain or chronic fatigue, or we just feel "off".

It might get more difficult to wake up in the morning, or it may be more difficult for us to go to sleep or to stay asleep at night. We may fidget, cannot focus, and feel anxious.

The autonomics also control many small functions like our pupil's ability to respond to bright sunlight without needing sunglasses, being able to see while driving at night, sweating, and temperature regulation.

When the autonomics malfunction it can makes us feel too hungry and contributes to obesity due to the false need to snack during the day for what we believe are "low blood sugar" symptoms. It can also produce abnormal hunger a few hours after having a full meal and stress hormones that contribute to stubborn belly fat.

Early autonomic dysfunction in adults includes high blood pressure, sleep apnea or insomnia, and cerebral blood flow issues that leave them with ADD, dizziness, brain fog, memory problems and anxiety.

Today's young adults and children are also experiencing a great deal of autonomic dysfunction. They are increasingly unable to heal from concussions, they have gastrointestinal and digestion trouble, and they are developing ADD/ADHD, autism, and anxiety.

Learning about the signs and stages of autonomic dysfunction may help you finally get to the underlying cause of your medical issues and provide a framework for you to regain your health.

Improving and reversing autonomic dysfunction is important for people of all ages because when the autonomics malfunction long enough, the resulting metabolic inflammation will ultimately help to turn on someone's genetics for disease.

Combining my 30 years of internal medicine expertise with autonomic nervous system analysis and an in-depth understanding of cell function and inflammation, I have developed treatment methods for preventing, reducing, or reversing acute and chronic autonomic nervous system damage.

WHAT IS THE AUTONOMIC NERVOUS SYSTEM?

The autonomic nervous system is the main communications network between the brain and the heart, the organs, the digestive tract, the lungs, and as well as immune system and hormonal regulation.

When your autonomics work correctly they are "automatic" and you do not even know they exist. The autonomics encompass almost everything that goes wrong when your body is not working "automatically" perfect like it should.

The nerves within the autonomics are the brain's master control mechanism for the body. The autonomics are not a new area of medicine, but until recently autonomics were only explored in research studies and labs, more fascinating to watch than practical in fighting common or complex illnesses.

The autonomic branches were also too complex to be tested in regular outpatient settings, and doctors did not know how to repair them once broken. But now advances in technology are making autonomic testing available in regular medical offices like mine, and I have discovered treatment methods for autonomic improvement or repair without long term medications.

The autonomics control every organ in the body such as the heart, bladder, stomach, intestines and kidneys. It is how the brain regulates your blood pressure, blood sugar, sleep cycles, immune system, and hormones.

The autonomics also control many smaller functions like when your pupils dilate, hiccups, and the adrenaline that produces nightmares. It controls basic bodily functions that no one really thinks about until the moment they start to malfunction.

The autonomics also coordinate our emotionality and how intensely we react to stressors, and they are tied to the cellular damage that creates anxiety, depression, PTSD, and autonomic disorders.

HOW DOES THE AUTONOMIC NERVOUS SYSTEM WORK?

The autonomic nervous system communicates and coordinates the metabolic state of the cells in the human body through two main branches. One is the sympathetic nervous system (sympathetic) and the other is the parasympathetic nervous system (parasympathetic).

In simple terms, the sympathetic branch is responsible for energy expenditure ("fight or flight") and the parasympathetic branch is responsible for energy conservation and restoration ("rest and digest").

The sympathetic branch controls the body's response to stress, pain, and cold. The parasympathetic branch controls the body's resting state after a meal, at night, the digestive tract, nutrient storage, immune responses, and healing.

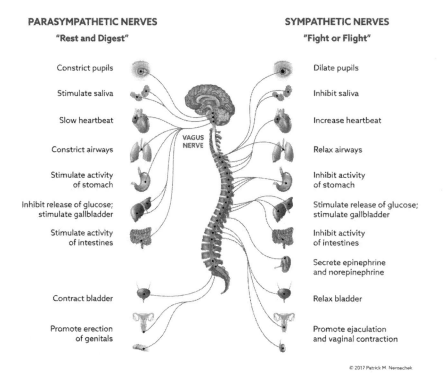

PARASYMPATHETIC NERVES
"Rest and Digest"

SYMPATHETIC NERVES
"Fight or Flight"

Parasympathetic	Sympathetic
Constrict pupils	Dilate pupils
Stimulate saliva	Inhibit saliva
Slow heartbeat	Increase heartbeat
Constrict airways	Relax airways
Stimulate activity of stomach	Inhibit activity of stomach
Inhibit release of glucose; stimulate gallbladder	Stimulate release of glucose; stimulate gallbladder
Stimulate activity of intestines	Inhibit activity of intestines
	Secrete epinephrine and norepinephrine
Contract bladder	Relax bladder
Promote erection of genitals	Promote ejaculation and vaginal contraction

VAGUS NERVE

© 2017 Patrick M. Nemechek

If the sympathetic commands are disrupted people may feel tired, crave salt or sugar, experience excessive hunger, or get anxious. People may get heart palpitations, tingling or numbness in their arms (hands or face), disrupted night vision, varicose veins, erectile dysfunction, stiff necks and shoulders, or severe ("migraine") headaches. Sympathetic dysfunction may also create adrenaline rushes that fuel insomnia, nightmares, aggression, or anger.

If the parasympathetic commands are disrupted they may affect the intestinal tract (heartburn or constipation), the immune system (autoimmune disorders), or produce chronic pain syndromes (fibromyalgia).

These people may get sleep apnea, "restless legs", morning nausea, night sweats or hot flashes, intolerance to light because of dilated pupils, or feel power surge sensations when they should be at rest. Parasympathetic dysfunction may leave them exhausted in the morning despite a full night of sleep.

Both the sympathetic and parasympathetic branches feed into the heart and modulate the heart's natural rhythms and ability for the heart muscle to contract.

Damage or disruption to the function of either of these branches causes a wide variety of symptoms to occur, and many people experience both sympathetic and parasympathetic branch symptoms.

These two opposite autonomic branches should work together simultaneously and in balance, which is called sympathovagal balance. When these two autonomic branches are in balance the body works automatically and a person feels no symptoms.

Without proper balance one branch may become withdrawn or the other becomes elevated. When the branches are no longer working automatically, a person may feel symptoms that range from mild (feeling dizzy or a getting a head rush when standing up from a chair) to completely debilitating (falling or passing out).

Sympathovagal balance between the sympathetic and parasympathetic branches is not just important for feeling better in the short term, sympathovagal balance is necessary for a long and healthy life.

My goal as a physician is to improve and restore autonomic functioning because it is critical to life expectancy. Improved autonomic function improves heart rate variability (HRV). People with elevated HRV have an increased risk of developing atrial fibrillation or heart flutter. People with low HRV have an increased risk of widespread organ and metabolic dysfunction.

When the sympathetic and parasympathetic branches are not in sympathovagal balance, and if left untreated, the imbalance will result in a loss of heart rate variability (HRV) which is associated with increased mortality from all causes.

Autonomic dysfunction also fuels the systemic metabolic inflammation that triggers cellular changes and ignites someone's disposition for disease (cancer, diabetes, hypertension, etc.).

WHAT ARE SOME CAUSES OF AUTONOMIC DYSFUNCTION?

The autonomic nervous system may be injured in a variety of ways:

- Head Injury (concussions)
- Emotional Trauma (intense emotional events, emotional concussions)
- Metabolic Injury (medications, chemo or radiation, heat stroke, alcohol intoxication)
- Inflammatory Injury (infections, tobacco smoke, excessive omega-6 fatty acid intake, vaccines, surgery, autoimmunity, allergy tests or allergy shots)
- Intestinal Bacterial Overgrowth (SIBO, dysbiosis)
- Pregnancy

HOW DOES RECOVERY OF AUTONOMIC DYSFUNCTION OCCUR?

I have found that the improvement and recovery of autonomic dysfunction is possible by inducing the nervous system and organs to repair themselves by normalizing inflammation control mechanisms, inducing natural stem cell production, and reactivating innate restorative mechanisms.

Recovery from autonomic dysfunction is a realistic goal and it can occur even decades after the injuries began.

- Symptoms Lessen as the Brain Repairs

- Core Nutrients Lower Brain Inflammation
- Stem Cell Production Resumes
- Natural Brain Repair Mechanisms Activate
- Vagus Nerve Stimulation Speeds Recovery (Adults)
- Cell Functions Normalize
- Long Term Damage is Reversible

THE FIVE STAGES OF AUTONOMIC DYSFUNCTION

Autonomic dysfunction occurs when the nerves that carry information from the brain to the heart, bladder, intestines, sweat glands, pupils, and blood vessels no longer function properly.

This improper function may affect different organ systems in different people, so symptoms may vary greatly from one person to the next person.

This improper function may also affect multiple systems in one person at the same time, which accounts for a number of health problems that seem very different and unrelated but actually originate in this one area of the nervous system.

Your timelines of events and illnesses will begin to make sense once you understand that autonomic injury and inflammation causes a variety of symptoms, and then triggers diseases such as diabetes, cancer, heart failure, and Alzheimer's.

My treatment program, The Nemechek Protocol™ for Autonomic Recovery, puts these pieces together and treats the underlying cause. The first step is spectral analysis of the autonomic nervous system to determine the type and severity of your autonomic dysfunction.

Spectral analysis allows us to detect your sympathetic branch and parasympathetic patterns of damage. There are five stages of autonomic dysfunction that show up as different strengths of sympathetic and parasympathetic function. Your test results are a biomarker for your brain's overall health and ability to correctly run your body.

STAGES 1 AND 2

There are five stages in autonomic dysfunction. Stage One and Stage Two do not have noticeable symptoms yet these preclinical changes in brain function are detected during spectral analysis autonomic testing.

Identifying subtle changes in brain function allows me the opportunity to work with my patients to reverse the damage and to prevent future complications.

As autonomic dysfunction progresses into Stage Three, people become unable to compensate for their autonomic abnormalities and their ability to handle disease and stress becomes impaired.

STAGE 3

In Stage 3 of autonomic dysfunction people start to experience symptoms that affect their daily life. At this point, autonomic dysfunction causes people to experience things like heartburn, headaches, intestinal distress, dizziness, excessive hunger or thirst, anxiety, sexual dysfunction (women and men), or poor sleep.

The progression of autonomic dysfunction also brings the inability to control the blood pressure and heart rates (Atrial fibrillation or flutter, palpitations, POTS), affects the forward movement of the digestive tract, and proper breathing (sleep apnea).

People experience problems with their immune system, hormone levels, and organ function. People no longer bounce back from illnesses or injury and they may suffer from chronic fatigue or chronic pain.

As autonomic function declines and inflammation rises their symptoms may also be mental or emotional in nature.

People have a harder time recovering from trauma and they may suffer from anxiety, panic attacks, depression, postpartum depression, and PTSD.

STAGE 4

In Stage 4 of autonomic dysfunction, multiple systems in the body malfunction and people feel increasingly worse. Blood pressure or blood sugars get harder to regulate even with medications, and people have poor responses to other medical therapies.

As their heart, immune system and hormone systems malfunction, and as depression or anxiety increase, people turn to a variety of medical specialties searching for answers and diagnoses to explain the avalanche of brain and body dysfunction.

Worsening autonomic patterns of sympathetic and/or parasympathetic weakness at rest, also called Low Heart Rate Variability (low HRV) or Advanced Autonomic Dysfunction, disrupts their daily quality of life.

Low HRV leaves them at a higher risk of death from all causes because their body is unable to respond to things like pneumonia, cancer, and infections.

STAGE 5

Like Stages 1 and 2, the decline into Stage 5 of autonomic dysfunction may be silent but it is detected through autonomic spectral analysis. As the autonomics continue to malfunction, autonomic testing reveals weaker parasympathetic function and increased Low HRV (Heart Rate Variability).

The most advanced autonomic test patterns of weak parasympathetic function are Diabetic Autonomic Neuropathy (DAN), and then Cardiac Autonomic Neuropathy (CAN) which has a 50% mortality rate within five years.

The autonomics are so suppressed in Stage 5 that the person has difficulty at times, like when they are artificially asleep under anesthesia, which increases their risk of sudden cardiac death.

One of the most important things I have discovered is that all five stages of autonomic dysfunction are capable of improvement or repair, even decades after the autonomic injury. For 30 years, I have been willing to adopt and adapt any treatment approach that offers a chance to improve the health and well-being of my patients.

I am fortunate my education and experience with complex disease allows me to significantly impact peoples' lives. I am proud to say I have developed The Nemechek Protocol™ for Autonomic Recovery that improves the health of many after they had been told there were no other options available.

Karla and Her Headaches

Karla is a 42-year-old woman who was suffering from headaches that occurred almost daily but once or twice per week would become so severe they were incapacitating. The headaches seemed to begin shortly after waking and would worsen through the day. Sitting still while riding in a car or a plane seemed to make them worsen.

Before menstruation the headaches almost always increased in intensity and were often accompanied with anxiety, fatigue, brain fog, tightness of the neck and shoulders, and occasional numbness of the hands.

She has always had occasional mild headaches but they increased in intensity after having her gall bladder removed. Since then her headaches became much more frequent and severe, and interestingly she now had problems with occasional heartburn from bananas and coffee.

Karla's autonomic testing revealed severe underlying sympathetic dysfunction which makes it hard for the body to pump enough blood upwards into the head and neck region when someone is upright. Karla's neck and scalp pain are referred to as 'coat hanger pain' and are caused by an inadequate delivery of oxygen into the muscles of the neck and scalp.

Low blood pressure into the head and neck can also cause fatigue, poor cognition (i.e. brain fog, ADD, ADHD), anxiety, numbness of hands, face or neck (i.e., neuronal ischemia), fidgety behaviors (toe tapping, sitting cross legged or with a leg folded underneath, frequent changing of body position while seated) and the symptoms referred to as "low blood sugar".

These symptoms often begin after getting out of bed and worsen through the day. Sitting or standing still, becoming overheated, decreases in progesterone levels (pre-menstruation or menopause), and mild viral infections all can exacerbate the low blood pressure and symptoms.

Karla's previous mild headaches worsened after her gall bladder surgery because the stress of the surgery caused an inflammatory injury to her autonomic nervous system and triggered bacterial over-growth of the small intestine which caused the intestinal problems.

Karla had seen several health providers but it seems like her tests always came up normal and she walked away with a few prescriptions that were just meant to cover up her symptoms. She was frustrated because no one seems to be trying to find and fix the source of her problems.

Within two months of starting The Nemechek Protocol™ for Autonomic Recovery, Karla's headaches had dramatically decreased in frequency and intensity as had most of her other symptoms. The intestinal issues almost completely resolved within the first two weeks of treatment.

After six months Karla's autonomic testing had returned to normal, she has not had a headache within the last three months, and she only needs to take a simple and inexpensive regimen of supplements that she can buy from a variety of online retailers.

Her anxiety, fatigue, brain fog, tightness of the neck and shoulders, and numbness of the hands have all resolved as well.

APPENDIX II - CUMULATIVE BRAIN INJURY

UNDERSTANDING CUMULATIVE BRAIN INJURY

As discussed previously in this book, Mo-microglia are responsible for monitoring the health of the neurons within the brain.

If a neuron becomes damaged from a trauma such as a concussion, the Mo-microglia transform themselves into the anti-inflammatory tissue repairing M2-microglia.

The M2-microglia then set about repairing the injured neurons over the next several weeks to months. Once repaired, the M2-microglia then transform themselves back into their natural resting state as a Mo-microglia, and wait to start the process all over again when the next injury occurs.

Over your lifetime, your brain experiences common injuries from mild to concussive head injuries (sports, auto accidents, falls), intense emotional traumas (divorce, financial stress, bullying, molestation, fear), and inflammatory stress (vaccines, abdominal surgery, fractures, infections).

Each of these injuries can result in cellular damage that are ultimately repaired by the healthy Mo to M2 microglia repair process.

Unfortunately, the LPS that leaks through the gut and finds its way into the brain permanently changes this finely tuned repair process.

After entering the central nervous system, LPS causes a large number of M0-microglia to undergo an abnormal, permanent transformation into the pro-inflammatory M1-microglia.

The shift from the surveillance M0-microglia to the inflammatory, damage provoking M1-microglia is referred to as "priming" within the scientific literature.

The primed M1-microglia are unique in that they are immortal and never die, and start producing excessive amounts of inflammatory cytokines that create an unhealthy environment for brain repair and neuron function.

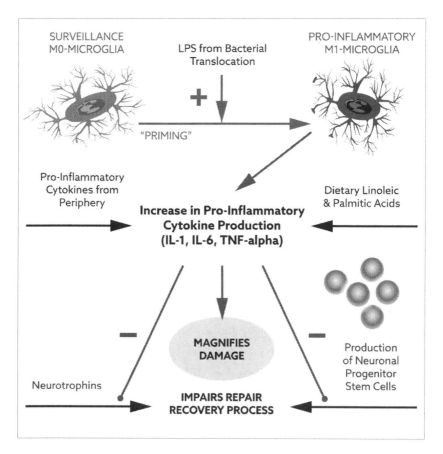

Excessive Pro-Inflammatory Cytokines within the Brain

With each subsequent injury, more and more M1-microglia are produced and inflammatory cytokines increase.

The combination results in magnifying the neuronal damage from each brain trauma. It also impairs stem cells from fully repairing that damage which leads to chronic brain damage from injuries that would have otherwise been fully reparable in a health, non-inflammatory brain.

Instead of injury and a complete recovery, a process of exaggerated damage and incomplete recovery begins. Each brain injury leaves behind a small residual brain defect, that is built upon by each subsequent injury through your life.

More damage and less recovery results in a process called cumulative brain injury (CBI).

The growing epidemic of chronic symptoms from unresolved concussion damage (known as post-concussion syndrome) is the direct result of an inflamed brain that is unable to repair itself from an injury.

Individuals with post-concussion syndrome often showed evidence of brain dysfunction prior to the triggering of a traumatic brain injury.

In other words, the athlete was already suffering from cumulative brain injury but was experiencing only mild symptoms that were not enough to impair their athletic performance.

It finally just takes one additional injury to push the athlete's cumulative damage beyond their ability to compensate and now they are given diagnoses such as dysautonomia, post-concussion syndrome, attention disorder (ADD/ADHD), or migraine headaches.

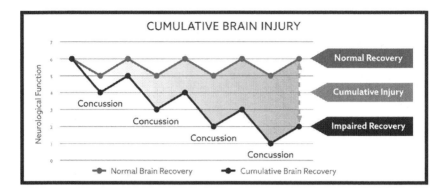

For non-athletically acquired cumulative brain injury, the neurological dysfunction may manifest in a wide array of common medical conditions such as whiplash, heartburn or reflux, irritable bowel syndrome (IBS), generalized anxiety disorder, chronic depression, chronic fatigue, postural orthostatic tachycardia syndrome (POTS), premenstrual syndrome (PMS) or menopause.

INFLAMMATORY CYTOKINES CONTRIBUTE TO CUMULATIVE BRAIN INJURY

In addition to primed microglia, pro-inflammatory cytokines are being chronically produced throughout your body from a wide array of sources which adds to the problem.

Cytokines are chemicals released from your white blood cells that change how other cells function. Cytokines that increase inflammation are produced as a result of excessive dietary linoleic acid intake (an omega-6 fatty acid found in many vegetable oils), a deficient intake of anti-inflammatory omega-3 fatty acids (found in fish oil, flax, nuts, wild game and fish), excessive dietary intake of AGEs (advanced glycation end products), abnormal stores of intra-abdominal fat, tobacco exposure, and the excessive consumption of carbohydrates, saturated fats, and calories in general.

Damage to the parasympathetic branch of the autonomic nervous system also causes a great deal of excessive inflammatory cytokine production as do most autoimmune disorders, surgeries, significant fractures, and treatments for cancer.

Inflammatory Cytokines are Produced By:

- Excessive Dietary Linoleic Acid (Omega-6)
- Deficient Intake of Omega-3 Fatty Acids
- Ingestion of AGEs (advanced glycation end products)
- Abnormal Stores Intra-Abdominal Fat
- Tobacco Use
- Secondhand Tobacco Exposure
- Excessive Carbohydrate Intake
- Excessive Saturated Fats Intake
- Excessive Calories Intake

These additional sources of inflammation only serve to worsen the brain's ability to repair itself and to maintain normal physical and emotional functioning.

If the pro-inflammatory cytokines reach high enough levels, they can result in the same cumulative brain injury process as microglia priming by LPS.

There is growing evidence that repeated head injuries (professional football, hockey, and soccer), significant imbalances of the ratio of omega-3 to omega-6 fatty acid dietary intake, and exposure to diesel fumes can initiate the permanent priming effect of microglia as well.

But how do the intestinal imbalance, increased inflammatory cytokine levels, and primed microglia affect a common person without a history of significant repetitive blows to the head?

AN EPIDEMIC OF UNRESOLVED CONCUSSIONS

Cumulative brain injury (CBI) is an almost invisible process because the type of injury causing the permanent damage (minor head trauma on a playground, the death of a loved one, or common vaccinations) have historically been understood to be harmless in the long run.

You go through life experiencing these events thinking that although unpleasant and difficult, you will fully recover and you will get on with your life. But as time goes on, you may begin noticing that you are developing some physical, emotional, or medical issues that you did not have before the injury or traumatic event.

You may start becoming a little more anxious, notice your headaches are more frequent, or that you now experience lightheadedness. You may notice your digestive system and response to foods are changing. Eating may seem to result in more and more heartburn or now constipation is making you feel uncomfortable.

And finally, you are being told your blood pressure and blood sugar numbers are rising, and you are placed on a variety of medications to control these conditions as well as some of your other symptoms.

You wonder how and why this happened. Part of the reason your health is changing is due to the cumulative brain injury you are experiencing from both traumatic and non-traumatic brain trauma.

You ask how you "caught" these medical problems. They seem to come out of nowhere without any explicable reason, but the truth is that they are originating in the bacterial imbalance of your intestinal tract along with other environmental factors that are adding to the building chemical inflammation in your body.

And due to the building chemical inflammation in your body, each new brain, physical, emotional, and inflammatory trauma now results in a growing amount of chronic dysfunction and damage to the autonomic nervous system and other areas of the brain.

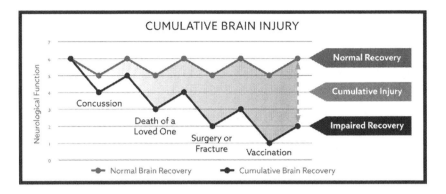

You have watched how your parents and grandparents have fearlessly dealt with these types of events because their life experience taught them as such. But things are much different than 50 years ago.

We are different. More and more of us are now suffering from bacterial imbalance and overgrowth and we are being mentally and physically affected by a growing number of sources of inflammation from our environment.

Eric, The Gulf War and PTSD

Eric is a 39-year-old man who had served as sergeant with the U.S. Marine Corp. during the Iraq War. He was involved in some very dangerous military action. He had been physically injured twice when the vehicles he was riding in were thrown in the air after being hit by explosives planted in the road.

Both events resulted in headaches and an altered sense of balance for a few weeks but those seemed to finally resolve. But what seemed to affect him the most was a fearful event when an enemy mortar round had landed four to five feet away from him, but it failed to fully discharge.

Eric heard what he described as "the loudest bang I've ever heard". When he saw the mortar-round stuck into the soil next to him he realized that he heard the detonating charge explode but the powerful and deadly explosive within the mortar had failed to ignite.

If it had done so, he understood quite clearly that he would have died.

Within a few minutes after this close call, Eric said he felt as if an emotional hammer struck him over the head. For a few weeks he felt emotionally numb, and this numbness turned into a severe depression.

He began having uncontrollable violent outbursts where he needed to physically destroy something.

He would smash a chair, a lamp, a window, anything that was at hand. He returned home but the depression and the destructive outbursts continued.

He went from job to job repeatedly being fired, not because his work performance, but because his destructive outbursts were incompatible with most workplace environments.

He was also suffering from chronic anxiety, heartburn, and frequent lightheadedness when getting out of bed or standing up.

Eric had been thoroughly evaluated by VA and community primary care physicians, neurologist, and psychiatrists. He was repeatedly diagnosed with post-traumatic stress disorder (PTSD) and generalized anxiety, and placed on medications.

The medications numbed him so much emotionally and cognitively that he stopped taking them except the medication to help with his sleep.

After his first visit with me he was excited to learn that new research is demonstrating that PTSD is the result of underlying cellular damage to areas of the brain called the hippocampus and the amygdala.

The hippocampus and the amygdala are known to control emotions, anxiety, and fear.

I explained that it was an inability of the brain to repair the damage to these areas that lead to the chronic nature of Eric's PTSD and anxiety, and that his light headedness was most likely the result of chronic damage to his autonomic nervous system from the concussions he suffered when the explosions flipped his vehicles upside down.

I explained that the military has published a few studies demonstrating the association between inflammation and PTSD as well as chronic autonomic damage.

Spectral analysis of Eric's autonomic nervous system demonstrated he had low heart rate variability (HRV) and sympathetic branch damage responsible for his lightheadedness and some of his anxiety.

Low HRV is a result of the same inflammatory process in the brain that contributes to chronic PTSD and chronic depression.

Eric also demonstrated an autonomic pattern called Paradoxical Parasympathetic Syndrome which is commonly associated with central sleep apnea, restless leg syndrome, insomnia, and narcolepsy.

Eric was started on The Nemechek Protocol™ for Autonomic Recovery, and within two months his lightheadedness had resolved and he was surprised to feel like his mood was "lighter".

He wanted to play more with his two young sons, and found he was not isolating himself any longer from his co-workers.

By the sixth month he said he had not had an angry outburst in the past two months (he had been averaging one or two outbursts every week), he was able to discontinue the sleeping medicine because his insomnia was gone, and he was surprised to feel a sense of happiness for the first time since he was shipped out to fight in the Iraq War.

Eric remains on The Nemechek Protocol™ that strongly reduces his brain inflammation and normalizes microglia function by balancing omega fatty acids, maintaining a healthy balance of intestinal bacteria, and daily bioelectric Vagus nerve stimulation.

APPENDIX III - AUTONOMIC BRAIN QUIZ

TAKE THE AUTONOMIC BRAIN QUIZ

Studies indicate that 80% of chronic disease is caused by dysfunction of the autonomic nervous system. Autonomic dysfunction impairs the normal function of all organs (kidneys, liver, heart, circulation, intestines and bladder), the immune system, hormone production and your emotional balance.

Many common but disturbing symptoms are a sign of a larger problem, autonomic dysfunction. Many medical conditions such as diabetes, high blood pressure, gout, sleep apnea, chronic headaches or migraines, chronic fatigue, heart rhythm problems, heart burn, and chronic constipation have autonomic dysfunction as a central mechanism in their development.

Fortunately, there is a simple, painless test that accurately measures the health of your autonomic nervous system. If abnormalities are detected, new techniques have been developed to help the autonomic nervous system to recover.

Recovery and normalization of autonomic function often leads to a remarkable improvement and even complete reversal of the medical conditions listed above.

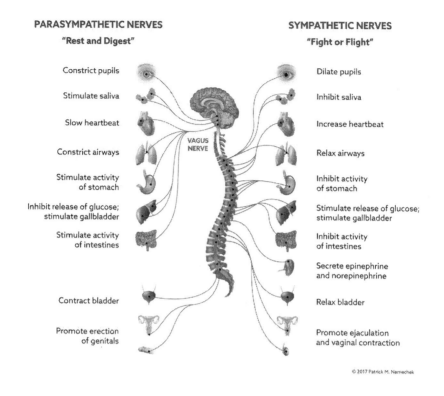

PARASYMPATHETIC NERVES
"Rest and Digest"

Constrict pupils

Stimulate saliva

Slow heartbeat

Constrict airways

Stimulate activity
of stomach

Inhibit release of glucose;
stimulate gallbladder

Stimulate activity
of intestines

Contract bladder

Promote erection
of genitals

VAGUS
NERVE

SYMPATHETIC NERVES
"Fight or Flight"

Dilate pupils

Inhibit saliva

Increase heartbeat

Relax airways

Inhibit activity
of stomach

Stimulate release of glucose;
stimulate gallbladder

Inhibit activity
of intestines

Secrete epinephrine
and norepinephrine

Relax bladder

Promote ejaculation
and vaginal contraction

© 2017 Patrick M. Nemechek

The Autonomic Nervous System

If your symptoms are lasting more than three months you may be developing chronic autonomic damage from cumulative brain injury.

If you have check more than three boxes you may have autonomic dysfunction.

Check the boxes that apply to you.

___ I am occasionally nauseated in the A.M.

___ I am dizzy or lightheaded at times.

___ I frequently feel anxious.

___ I have trouble with memory or concentration.

___ I feel unusually tired during the day.

___ I have "brain fog" at times.

___ I have trouble waking up in the morning.

___ I get frequent headaches or migraines.

___ I feel tightness in my neck or shoulder muscles.

___ I feel thirsty or hungry through the day.

___ My hands, face, or neck go numb periodically.

___ I find myself craving salt or sugar.

___ I become sleepy after a meal.

___ I frequently urinate.

___ I get heartburn or reflux.

___ I experience "PMS" before menstruation.

___ I have trouble sleeping.

___ I have difficulty getting an erection.

___ I have trouble seeing in bright or dim light.

___ I have passed out or fainted.

___ I feel weak when I get hot.

___ I have heart palpitations or an abnormal rhythm.

___ I feel excessively hot or cold.

___ My labs are fine but I feel "off".

CHECKING THREE OR MORE MEANS YOU MAY HAVE AUTONOMIC DYSFUNCTION

Researchers have studied the autonomic nervous system for decades but clinical autonomic medicine, which means using it in a primary care type setting, is new. Checking yes to the common symptoms of autonomic dysfunction may help you realize that the various symptoms represented in those boxes actually share common causes within the nervous system.

Autonomic testing via spectral analysis is a painless and rapid 17-minute test and provides critical information as to why you do not feel well. and this is the first step towards understanding how to make you feel healthy again.

As outlined in Appendix 1, autonomic dysfunction can be caused by the medications used in general anesthesia, an imbalance of intestinal bacteria, pregnancy, mild to severe concussions, emotionally traumatic events, an imbalance of dietary omega-6 and omega-3 fatty acid intake, and processed food.

APPENDIX IV - SCIENTIFIC REFERENCES

We have provided a sampling of the many research articles that have helped shape the development of The Nemechek Protocol™.

Autonomic Dysfunction:

- Bjørklund G. Cerebral hypoperfusion in autism spectrum disorder. Acta Neurobiol Expo (Wars). 2018;78(1):21-29. https://www.ncbi.nlm.nih.gov/pubmed/29694338
- Goodman B. Autonomic Dysfunction in Autism Spectrum Disorders (ASD). *Neurology* April 5, 2016 vol. 86 no. 16 Supplement P5.117. http://www.neurology.org/content/86/16_Supplement/P5.117
- Anderson CJ et al. Pupil and Salivary Indicators of Autonomic Dysfunction in Autism Spectrum Disorder. *Developmental psychobiology*. 2013;55(5):10.1002/dev.21051. https://www.ncbi.nlm.nih.gov/pmc/articles/PMC3832142/

- Goodman B et al. Autonomic Nervous System Dysfunction in Concussion. *Neurology* February 12, 2013 vol. 80 no. 7 Supplement P01.265. http://www.neurology.org/content/80/7_Supplement/P01.265

- La Fountaine MF. et al. Autonomic Nervous System Responses to Concussion: Arterial Pulse Contour Analysis. *Frontiers in Neurology* 7 (2016): 13. https://www.ncbi.nlm.nih.gov/pmc/articles/PMC4756114/

- Amhed K. Assessment of Autonomic Function in Children with Autism and Normal Children Using Spectral Analysis and Posture Entrainment: A Pilot Study. *J of Neurology and Neuroscience*. 2015. Vol. 6 No. 3:37. http://www.jneuro.com/neurology-neuroscience/assessment-of-autonomic-function-in-children-with-autism-and-normal-children-using-spectral-analysis-and-posture-entrainment-a-pilot-study.pdf

Bacterial Overgrowth:

- Adams JB et al. Gastrointestinal flora and gastrointestinal status in children with autism -- comparisons to typical children and correlation with autism severity. *BMC Gastroenterology*. 2011. https://www.ncbi.nlm.nih.gov/pubmed/21410934

- Wang L. Hydrogen breath test to detect small intestinal bacterial overgrowth: a prevalence case control study in autism. *Eur Child Adolesc Psychiatry*. 2017 Aug 10. https://www.ncbi.nlm.nih.gov/pubmed/28799094

- Hsiao EY et al. The microbiota modulates gut physiology and behavioral abnormalities associated with autism. *Cell*. 2013;155(7):1451-1463. https://www.ncbi.nlm.nih.gov/pmc/articles/PMC3897394/

- Cryan JF et al. Mind-altering microorganisms: the impact of the gut microbiota on brain and behaviour. *Nat Rev Neurosci.* 2012 Oct;13(10):701-12.
  https://www.ncbi.nlm.nih.gov/pubmed/22968153

Cumulative Brain Injury:

- Cunningham C. Microglia and neurodegeneration: the role of systemic inflammation. *J Neurosci.* 2013 Mar 6;33(10):4216-33.
  https://www.ncbi.nlm.nih.gov/pubmed/22674585
- Wager-Smith, Karen, and Athina Markou. Depression: A Repair Response to Stress-Induced Neuronal Microdamage That Can Grade into a Chronic Neuroinflammatory Condition?*Neuroscience and biobehavioral reviews* 35.3 (2011): 742–764.
  https://www.ncbi.nlm.nih.gov/pubmed/20883718

Histamine:

- Visciano P et al. Biogenic Amines in Raw and Processed Seafood. *Frontiers in Microbiology.* 2012;3:188.
  https://www.ncbi.nlm.nih.gov/pmc/articles/PMC3366335/
- Feng c et al. Histamine (Scombroid) Fish Poisoning: a Comprehensive Review. *Clin Rev Allergy Immunol.* 2016 Feb;50(1):64-9.
  https://www.ncbi.nlm.nih.gov/pubmed/25876709
- Jin X et al. Increased intestinal permeability in pathogenesis and progress of nonalcoholic steatohepatitis in rats. *World Journal of Gastroenterology: WJG.* 2007;13(11):1732-1736.
  https://www.ncbi.nlm.nih.gov/pubmed/17461479
- Guo Y et al. Functional changes of intestinal mucosal

barrier in surgically critical patients. *World Journal of Emergency Medicine.* 2010;1(3):205-208. https://www.ncbi.nlm.nih.gov/pmc/articles/PMC4129678/

Inulin:

- Kellow NJ et al. Effect of dietary prebiotic supplementation on advanced glycation, insulin resistance and inflammatory biomarkers in adults with pre-diabetes: a study protocol for a double-blind placebo-controlled randomized crossover clinical trial. *BMC Endocrine Disorders.* 2014;14:55. https://www.ncbi.nlm.nih.gov/pubmed/25011647
- Hopkins MJ, Macfarlane GT. Nondigestible Oligosaccharides Enhance Bacterial Colonization Resistance against *Clostridium difficile* In Vitro. *Applied and Environmental Microbiology.* 2003;69(4):1920-1927. https://www.ncbi.nlm.nih.gov/pmc/articles/PMC154806/
- Collins S, Reid G. Distant Site Effects of Ingested Prebiotics. *Nutrients.* 2016;8(9):523. https://www.ncbi.nlm.nih.gov/pmc/articles/PMC5037510/
- Slavin J. Significance of Inulin Fructans in the Human Diet. *Compre Rev in Food Science and Food Safety.* 2015 14;1: 37–47. http://onlinelibrary.wiley.com/doi/10.1111/1541-4337.12119/abstract

Microglia and Neuroinflammation:

- Petrelli F, Pucci L, Bezzi P. Astrocytes and Microglia and Their Potential Link with Autism Spectrum Disorders. *Frontiers in Cellular Neuroscience.* 2016;10:21. https://www.ncbi.nlm.nih.gov/pmc/articles/PMC4751265/

- Norden, DM et al. Microglial Priming and Enhanced Reactivity to Secondary Insult in Aging, and Traumatic CNS Injury, and Neurodegenerative Disease. *Neuropharmacology* 96.0 0 (2015): 29–41. https://www.ncbi.nlm.nih.gov/pmc/articles/PMC4430467/
- Calabrese, F et al. Brain-Derived Neurotrophic Factor: A Bridge between Inflammation and Neuroplasticity. *Frontiers in Cellular Neuroscience* 8 (2014): 430. https://www.ncbi.nlm.nih.gov/pmc/articles/PMC4273623/
- Cunningham, Colm. Systemic Inflammation and Delirium – Important Co-Factors in the Progression of Dementia. *Biochemical Society Transactions* 39.4 (2011): 945–953. https://www.ncbi.nlm.nih.gov/pubmed/21787328
- Paolicelli RC et al. Synaptic pruning by microglia is necessary for normal brain development. *Science* 2011 Sep 9;333(6048):1456-8. https://www.ncbi.nlm.nih.gov/pubmed/21778362

Omega Fatty Acids:

- Madsen L, Kristiansen K. Of mice and men: Factors abrogating the anti-obesity effect of omega-3 fatty acids. *Adipocyte.* 2012;1(3):173-176. https://www.ncbi.nlm.nih.gov/pmc/articles/PMC3609096/
- El-Ansary AK et al. On the protective effect of omega-3 against propionic acid-induced neurotoxicity in rat pups. *Lipids in Health and Disease.* 2011;10:142. https://www.ncbi.nlm.nih.gov/pmc/articles/PMC3170231/
- Chang, P et al. Docosahexaenoic Acid (DHA): A Modulator of Microglia Activity and Dendritic Spine Morphology. *Journal of Neuroinflammation* 12 (2015): 34. https://www.ncbi.nlm.nih.gov/pmc/articles/PMC4344754/

- Patterson E et al. Health Implications of High Dietary Omega-6 Polyunsaturated Fatty Acids. *Journal of Nutrition and Metabolism.* 2012;2012:539426. https://www.ncbi.nlm.nih.gov/pubmed/22570770
- Harvey, LD. et al. Administration of DHA Reduces Endoplasmic Reticulum Stress-Associated Inflammation and Alters Microglial or Macrophage Activation in Traumatic Brain Injury. *ASN Neuro* 7.6 (2015): 1759091415618969. https://www.ncbi.nlm.nih.gov/pmc/articles/PMC4710127/
- Liu, JJ. et al. Pathways of Polyunsaturated Fatty Acid Utilization: Implications for Brain Function in Neuropsychiatric Health and Disease. *Brain research* 0 (2015): 220–246. https://www.ncbi.nlm.nih.gov/pmc/articles/PMC4339314/
- Titos E et al. Resolvin D1 and its precursor docosahexaenoic acid promote resolution of adipose tissue inflammation by eliciting macrophage polarization toward an M2-like phenotype. *J Immun.* 2011 Nov 15;187(10):5408-18. https://www.ncbi.nlm.nih.gov/pubmed/22013115
- Chen S et al. n-3 PUFA supplementation benefits microglial responses to myelin pathology. *Scientific Reports.* 2014;4:7458. https://www.ncbi.nlm.nih.gov/pubmed/25500548
- Minkyung K et al. Impact of 8-week linoleic acid intake in soy oil on Lp-PLA2 activity in healthy adults. *Nutr & Metab.* 2017. 14:32. https://www.ncbi.nlm.nih.gov/pmc/articles/PMC5422895/
- Christian LM et al. Body weight affects ω-3 polyunsaturated fatty acid (PUFA) accumulation in youth following supplementation in post-hoc analyses of a randomized controlled trial. *PLoS ONE.* 2017;12(4):e0173087. https://www.ncbi.nlm.nih.gov/pmc/articles/PMC5381773/

- Igarashi M et al. Dietary N-6 Polyunsaturated Fatty Acid Deprivations Increases Docosahexaenoic Acid (DHA) in Rat Brain. *Journal of Neurochemistry.* 2012;120(6):985-997. https://www.ncbi.nlm.nih.gov/pmc/articles/PMC3296886/
- Grundy T et al. Long-term omega-3 supplementation modulates behavior, hippocampal fatty acid concentration, neuronal progenitor proliferation and central TNF-α expression in 7 month old unchallenged mice. *Frontiers in Cellular Neuroscience.* 2014;8:399. https://www.ncbi.nlm.nih.gov/pmc/articles/PMC4240169/

Prevention:

- Chu DM et al. Maturation of the Infant Microbiome Community Structure and Function Across Multiple Body Sites and in Relation to Mode of Delivery. *Nature medicine.* 2017;23(3):314-326. https://www.ncbi.nlm.nih.gov/pubmed/28112736
- Arslanoglu S et al. Early supplementation of prebiotic oligosaccharides protects formula-fed infants against infections during the first 6 months of life. *J Nutr.* 2007 Nov;137(11):2420-4. https://www.ncbi.nlm.nih.gov/pubmed/17951479
- Helland IB et al. Maternal supplementation with very-long-chain n-3 fatty acids during pregnancy and lactation augments children's IQ at 4 years of age. *Pediatrics.* 2003 Jan;111(1):e39-44. https://www.ncbi.nlm.nih.gov/pubmed/12509593
- Desai et al. Depletion of Brain Docosahexaenoic Acid Impairs Recovery from Traumatic Brain Injury. Annunziato L, ed. *PLoS ONE.* 2014;9(1):e86472. https://www.ncbi.nlm.nih.gov/pubmed/24475126
- Carlson SE et al. DHA supplementation and pregnancy

outcomes. *The American Journal of Clinical Nutrition.* 2013;97(4):808-815.
https://www.ncbi.nlm.nih.gov/pubmed/23426033

- Carvajal JA. Docosahexaenoic Acid Supplementation Early in Pregnancy May Prevent Deep Placentation Disorders. *BioMed Research International.* 2014;2014:526895.
https://www.ncbi.nlm.nih.gov/pubmed/25019084

- Fukuda H et al. Inhibition of sympathetic pathways restores postoperative ileus in the upper and lower gastrointestinal tract. *J Gastroenterol Hepatol.* 2007 Aug; 22(8):12939.
https://www.ncbi.nlm.nih.gov/pubmed/17688668

- Perring S et al. Assessment of changes in cardiac autonomic tone resulting from inflammatory response to the influenza vaccination. *Clin Physiol Funct Imaging.* 2012 Nov;32(6):437-44.
https://www.ncbi.nlm.nih.gov/pubmed/23031064

- Jae SY et al. Does an acute inflammatory response temporarily attenuate parasympathetic reactivation? *Clin Auton Res.* 2010 Aug;20(4):229-33.
https://www.ncbi.nlm.nih.gov/pubmed/20437076

- De Wildt DJ et al. Impaired autonomic responsiveness of the cardiovascular system of the rat induced by a heat-labile component of Bordetella pertussis vaccine. *Infection and Immunity.* 1983;41(2):476-481.
https://www.ncbi.nlm.nih.gov/pmc/articles/PMC264665/

- Kashiwagi Y et al. Production of inflammatory cytokines in response to diphtheria-pertussis-tetanus (DPT), *haemophilus influenzae* type b (Hib), and 7-valent pneumococcal (PCV7) vaccines. *Human Vaccines & Immunotherapeutics.* 2014;10(3):677-685.
https://www.ncbi.nlm.nih.gov/pmc/articles/PMC4130255/

- Akiho H et al. Cytokine-induced alterations of gastrointestinal motility in gastrointestinal

disorders. *World Journal of Gastrointestinal Pathophysiology.* 2011;2(5):72-81.
https://www.ncbi.nlm.nih.gov/pmc/articles/PMC3196622/

- Vantrappen G et al. The Interdigestive Motor Complex of Normal Subjects and Patients with Bacterial Overgrowth of the Small Intestine. *Journal of Clinical Investigation.* 1977;59(6):1158-1166.
https://www.ncbi.nlm.nih.gov/pmc/articles/PMC372329/

- Jacobs C et al. Dysmotility and PPI use are independent risk factors for small intestinal bacterial and/or fungal overgrowth. *Alimentary pharmacology & therapeutics.* 2013;37(11):1103-1111.
https://www.ncbi.nlm.nih.gov/pmc/articles/PMC3764612/

- Miyano Y et al. The Role of the Vagus Nerve in the Migrating Motor Complex and Ghrelin- and Motilin-Induced Gastric Contraction in Suncus. Covasa M, ed. *PLoS ONE.* 2013;8(5):e64777.
https://www.ncbi.nlm.nih.gov/pmc/articles/PMC3665597/

Propionic Acid and Autism:

- El-Ansary AK et al. Etiology of autistic features: the persisting neurotoxic effects of propionic acid. *Journal of Neuroinflammation.* 2012;9:74.
https://www.ncbi.nlm.nih.gov/pubmed/22531301

- McFabe DF et al. Neurobiological effects of intraventricular propionic acid in rats possible role of short chain fatty acids on the pathogenesis and characteristics of autism spectrum disorders. *Behav Brain Res.* 2007. Jan 10:176(1);149-69.
https://www.ncbi.nlm.nih.gov/pubmed/16950524

- Xiong X, Liu D, Wang Y, Zeng T, Peng Y. Urinary 3-(3-Hydroxyphenyl)-3-hydroxypropionic Acid, 3-

Hydroxyphenylacetic Acid, and 3-Hydroxyhippuric Acid Are Elevated in Children with Autism Spectrum Disorders. *BioMed Research International.* 2016. https://www.ncbi.nlm.nih.gov/pmc/articles/PMC4829699/

- MacFabe DF. Short-chain fatty acid fermentation products of the gut microbiome: implications in autism spectrum disorders. *Microbial Ecology in Health and Disease.* 2012;23:10. https://www.ncbi.nlm.nih.gov/pubmed/23990817

Rifaximin:

- Ponziani FR et al. Eubiotic properties of rifaximin: Disruption of the traditional concepts in gut microbiota modulation. *World Journal of Gastroenterology.* 2017;23(25):4491-4499. https://www.ncbi.nlm.nih.gov/pmc/articles/PMC3747729/
- Gao, J et al. Rifaximin, gut microbes and mucosal inflammation: unraveling a complex relationship. Gut Microbes. 2014 Jul 1;5(4):571-5. https://www.ncbi.nlm.nih.gov/pubmed/25244596
- Yao CK. The clinical value of breath hydrogen testing. *J Gastroenterologists Hepatol.* 2017 Mar;32 Suppl 1:20-22. https://www.ncbi.nlm.nih.gov/pubmed/28244675
- Ghoshal UC et al. Utility of hydrogen breath tests in diagnosis of small intestinal bacterial overgrowth in malabsorption syndrome and its relationship with orocecal transit time. *Indian J Gastroenterol.* 2006 Jan-Feb;25(1):6-10. https://www.ncbi.nlm.nih.gov/pmc/articles/PMC4175689/
- Muniyappa P et al. Use and safety of rifaximin in children with inflammatory bowel disease. *J Pediatricians Gastroenterol Nutr.* 2009 Oct;49(4):400-4. https://www.ncbi.nlm.nih.gov/pubmed/19668011

- Pimentel M, Cash BD, Lembo A, Wolf RA, Israel RJ, Schoenfeld P. Repeat Rifaximin for Irritable Bowel Syndrome: No Clinically Significant Changes in Stool Microbial Antibiotic Sensitivity. *Digestive Diseases and Sciences.* 2017;62(9):2455-2463. https://www.ncbi.nlm.nih.gov/pmc/articles/PMC5561162/

READER'S NOTES

-
  -
  -
  -
  -
  -
  -
  -
  -
  -
  -
  -
  -
  -
  -
  -
  -
  -
  -
  -

-
-
-
-
-
-
-
-
-
-
-
-
-
-
-
-
-
-
-
-
-
-
-
-
-
-
-
-
-
-
-
-
-

-
-
-
-
-
-
-
-
-
-
-
-
-
-
-
-
-
-
-
-
-
-
-
-
-
-
-
-
-
-
-
-
-

PROJECTS IN DEVELOPMENT

- The Nemechek Protocol™ - A Guide for Recovery from Adult Cumulative Brain Injuries
- The Autonomic Advantage™ Brain Injury Recovery Program for Athletes
- The Nemechek Protocol™ Practitioner Certification Program
- The Autonomic Advantage™ Training Course for Autonomic Assessment, Interpretation and Clinical Management
- The Nemechek Protocol™ Monitoring App

For more information about certification and licensing:
Info@AutonomicMed.com

Additional Resources:
AutonomicMed.com
AutonomicRecovery.com
@ConcussionFixer
https://www.youtube.com/user/pnemechek

Made in the USA
Middletown, DE
04 October 2020